Miracle Cure: Organic Germanium

DISTRIBUTED BY:
BIOCURRENTS PRESS
DIVISION OF NUTRI-COLOGY INC.
P. O. BOX 306
SAN LEANDRO, CA 94577
(415) 639 - 4572
COST: $17.95

Miracle Cure
Organic Germanium

Kazuhiko Asai, Ph. D.

 Japan Publications, Inc.

This book is dedicated to Hiroshi Oikawa, Sc. D., who devoted himself to the research on Germanium for 30 years together with me, and, my wife and four children who shared joys and sorrows with me.

© 1980 by Kazuhiko Asai

All rights reserved. No part of this publication may be reproduced, stored in a retrieval system, or transmitted, in any form or by any means, electronic, mechanical photocopying, recording or otherwise, without the prior written permission of the publisher.

Published by JAPAN PUBLICATIONS, INC., Tokyo & New York

Distributors:
UNITED STATES: *Kodansha International/USA, Ltd., through Harper & Row, Publishers, Inc., 10 East 53rd Street, New York, 10022.* SOUTH AMERICA: *Harper & Row, Publishers, Inc., International Department.* CANADA: *Fitzhenry & Whiteside Ltd., 195 Allstate Parkway, Markham, Ontario, L3R 4T8.* MEXICO AND CENTRAL AMERICA: *HARLA S. A. de C. V., Apartado 30–546, Mexico 4, D. F.* BRITISH ISLES: *International Book Distributors Ltd., 66 Wood Lane End, Hemel Hempstead, Herts HP2 4RG.* EUROPEAN CONTINENT: *Fleetbooks-Feffer and Simons (Nederland), 61 Strijkviertel, 3454 PK de Meern, The Netherlands.* AUSTRALIA AND NEW ZEALAND: *Bookwise International, 1 Jeanes Street, Beverley, South Australia 5007.* THE FAR EAST AND JAPAN: *Japan Publications Trading Co., Ltd., 1-2-1, Sarugaku-cho, Chiyoda-ku, Tokyo 101.*

First edition: November 1980
Second printing: February 1987

LCCC No. 79–91512
ISBN 0–87040–474–1

Printed in U.S.A.

Preface

Arthur Kestler in his book entitled *The Intrinsic Nature of Change*, offers this conclusion. It is futile to try to arrive at an understanding or a solution of the "intrinsic nature of chance" by conventional scientific common sense. The thing to do is to postulate that chance, which is of a higher dimension than the four-dimensional world, exists and to think that the postulate is an actuality. In short, chance is beyond understanding by conventional scientific common sense but it really does exist. Inevitability of chance may be an apt description. With regard to procreation and genesis of living things, particularly of human beings, for instance, the probability of the births of males and females should mathematically be 100 to 100. Actually, however, the ratio is 106 males to 100 females. Therein lies the inevitability arising from the mysterious rationality of nature.

My connection with germanium started by chance, certainly, but I cannot help perceiving there a working of some supernormal inevitability. If I may be permitted to express unhesitatingly my sensibility and fidelity to my thinking, I believe that my life is inextricably linked with germanium and that my germanium compound was divinely conferred on mankind through an actual being; that being happened to be I.

It may have been presumptuous of me, but I have endeavored, from beginning to end, ultimately to suggest some unknown laws existing in the universe by interweaving emotional expressions among the intellectual contents presented as the main body of this book. When I review the seventy-odd years of my life, I seem to find a consistent thread or a command from some outside source that transcends my own will which has determined my continued research of this amazing compound.

Though I have not received a formal education in the field of modern medicine, I believe I have ample reverence for human life. The very essence of the healing arts must find its basis in the great premise of life itself. In other words, its substance must be a religious-like concept of saving the sick. Through germanium I have come to know the thrill of living. I want to experience that by forgetting myself and saving others. My encounter with germanium was indeed by chance but it is a substance understandable only through high level meditative deliberations with a highly sharpened mind.

All my years of study with germanium have led me to know the wonderful action the germanium compound can have among all people. To disseminate this precious knowledge, without hesitation or timidity I raise my voice in praise of germanium. I hope that this small voice can reach the hearts of all my fellowmen. I have written in narrative style of my experience with germanium, and in order to penetrate the hearts and minds of men I have made use of some fables and parables, but all is genuine and based solely on fact.

When I gaze upon the single crystal of germanium with its silver-gray sheen, I have the illusion of seeing my whole life crystallized in this substance; I also feel, on the palm of my hand, the touch of a substance I am tempted to describe as the fountain of life that fills the universe.

Kazuhiko Asai, Ph.D.

A Biographical Sketch of Kazuhiko Asai

Dr. Kazuhiko Asai was born on the 30th of March, 1908 as the eldest son of Masajiro Asai who was working at that time as an educator of Chinese pupils in Dairen, Manchuria, the northeastern province of China. He stayed there until he was 10 years old; after that the family moved to Tokyo, where he graduated from the Imperial University of Tokyo, Faculty Jurisprudence, in 1932.

In the spring of 1934 he was sent to Berlin as the representative of Okura Trading Co., Ltd. He matriculated at the polytechnium in Charlottenburg, Berlin, in 1940, where he studied mining and metallurgy, for four years. He stayed in Berlin till its fall to the Russian army in 1945.

He returned to Japan in July 1945 and established the Coal Research Institute, where he studied with several assistants the nature of coal in Japan. The institute has been instrumental in introducing steel beams and columns to replace wooden beams and columns in coal mines in this country. His research at the institute led to the discovery of germanium in coal and the extraction of germanium from coal gas waste liquid.

In 1953 he represented Japan at the International Congress on the Study of Coal Structure. The same year he was appointed to teach the subject of coal petrology at the Second Engineering Department at Tokyo University and at the Science Faculty of Kyushu University.

In 1957, he was awarded the Purple Order of Merit for his various achievements in the field of technical development.

In 1962 a doctorate for technology by the University of Kyoto was conferred on him.

In 1967 he received an award by the Fuel Association.

In 1969 the Asai Germanium Research Institute was established.

In January 1975 he was elected a member of the New York Academy of Science.

At present he continues his research and directs the Organic Germanium Clinic (6-4-13, Seijo, Setagaya-ku, Tokyo, Japan: Telephone 03(482) 0590, 0690).

Dr. Asai is married to Erika (née Hoelterhof) and has a son and three daughters.

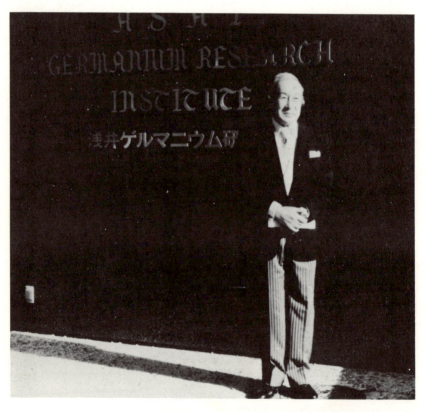

Kazuhiko Asai, Ph.D.

Contents

Preface
A Biographical Sketch of Kazuhiko Asai

Introduction

Biological Significance of Germanium
 1. The Element Germanium: Historical Background, 17
 2. Germanium: A Semiconductor, 18
 3. The Existence of Germanium in Coal, 19
 4. Germanium and Plants, 22
 5. A Weapon for Self-defense, 25
 6. Synthesis of Organic Germanium Compound, 29
 7. Myself as the Living Body Test, 31
 8. Effects on Animals, 34
 9. Germanium as an Experimental Medicine, 35
 10. Mechanism of Action, 37
 11. Substitute for Oxygen, 38

Germanium and Health
 1. Well-Balanced Diet, Prerequisite to Good Health, 41
 2. Pregnancy, 43
 3. Birth of Healing Life, 44
 4. Reasons for Oxygen Deficit in the Body, 48
 5. Stress, 49
 6. Elixir of Life, 51

Germanium in the Treatment of Disease in General
1. Methods of Treatment at the Clinic, 54
2. Excerpt from the Director's File of the Clinic, 55
3. Cases Taken from Clinic Records, 61
4. Two Examples Using Organic Germanium, 62
5. Efficacy on Eye Disease, 65
6. Efficacy on Hypertension 66
7. Effect of Germanium on Glands, 67
8. Experience with Organic Germanium: Dr. Takahiro Tanaka, 69
9. Experience with Organic Germanium: Dr. Okazawa, 72
10. Guarding against the Effects of Pollution, 81
11. Efficacy in Children, 84
12. Germanium and the Mind, 90
13. Treatment of Depressive Psychosis, 92
14. Attendance at the World Congress of Natural Medicine, 96
15. In Conclusion, 97

Germanium in the Treatment of Cancer
1. A Challenge to Cancer Cells, 99
2. Prevention of Metastasis, 103
3. Experiences with Lung and Prostate Gland Cancers, 104
4. In Praise of Germanium in Lung Cancer, 106
5. A Patient's Struggle with Cartilage Malignancy, 109
6. My Struggle with Cancer of the Larynx, 114
7. Germanium and Leukemia, 118
8. Death of a Widow, 121
9. Death of a Maiden, 124
10. Peaceful Death, 130
11. Concluding Remarks, 131

From the Logical World of Science to the Mystic World of God
1. Miracle Waters, 133
2. Water of Lourdes, 134
3. Yamabuki-no-Omizu (Mountain Rose Spring), 136

      4. Germanium Bathing, 139
      5. Religion, Divination and Germanium, 140

Future Trend in Medical Treatment—Inducement of the Body's Natural Healing Power

A Prayer for Germanium

    Appendix
    Index

Introduction

The tradition of Western medicine is now strong in Japan, and because I promulgate the theory of a common cause for all disease, I have incurred much opposition. Some doctors have even gone so far as to call for the eradication of this "amateur with no medical training who puts forth such irregular ideas." So, while hoping that germanium will bring about a radical change in the fundamental philosophy of life in the medical world, I am also aware that I am likely to be exposed to violent denunciations.

In the Germanium Clinic which I supervise, no pharmaceuticals are used, only my organic germanium. Therefore, when a patient comes to the Clinic he receives a medical examination and the appropriate prescription of germanium is given. In spite of the fact that no additional medicine is given, people come daily from all over Japan, and close to twenty per cent of them become so-called "germanium believers," continuing to take the compound over a long period. Of course, the purpose of the treatment has already been achieved, but repeated use has not once caused any side effects or any other complaint up to the present time, nor do I expect any in the future.

On the other hand, requests from practising physicians have greatly increased. Some of these doctors say that thanks to germanium, their patients are extremely grateful, and now without germanium they would be unable to continue their practice.

The effect of the compound is so unlike that of any medicine heretofore discovered that I hesitate to call germanium a medicine. I would rather call it a health-giving substance—i.e., a substance which restores a condition of health to those afflicted with disease, and which sustains a condition of health in those who are healthy. The basis for this, first, is its seemingly universal applicability and beneficial effect in the treatment of apparently any disease in adults and children. Secondly, it is without the adverse effects associated with medicines as we know them.

To my way of thinking there are three conditions for the treatment of disease which greatly affect recovery. These factors are supported by the latest advances in medical theory and endorsed by doctors working with the organic germanium compound. The principles of natural law form the basis for my thoughts and medical techniques, such as biorhythm, as well as acupuncture and natural herb therapy may be used in conjunction with them. The first condition for insuring the recovery of a person afflicted with disease is that he must have a firm conviction that he will recover. The expression "Heaven helps those who help themselves," should not be taken lightly. To a certain extent, the patient must become his own doctor in order to give full play to the healing powers of the body by personal involvement in the treatment. Underscoring this idea is the theory of electric potentials of a diseased organ as it relates to stress as a cause of disease. Just as stress can be said to cause cancer, ulcers, and other diseases, the stress or strain developed in these particles cannot be reversed if the strain is not eliminated by restoring harmony of the mind. Biorhythm healing methods rely on just this sort of harmony.

The second condition is the maintenance of proper diet. As mentioned previously, maximum effort should be made to maintain a balanced diet to prevent the blood from acidity, which happens if there is an excessive intake of hydrogen ions which consume the body oxygen and literally pollute the blood. The only way we can keep our blood clean and guarantee good health is by maintaining a proper acid-base balance. The third condition, a synthesis of the above two, is not a continuous combustion process to develop an oxygen deficiency. We remain alive because there is a continuous combustion process within the body to supply life-sustaining energy, a process in which oxygen plays the main role. If no effort is made to maintain a healthy mind and body by avoiding stress and an imbalanced diet, an oxygen deficiency will result.

The main factor involved in the curative effect of germanium then, is the life-style of the individual. Thus, on an individual basis success of treatment can be interpreted to be anywhere from 100% to 0, depending on how well the patient follows the conditions of treatment. Usually, disease is the result of an unbalanced diet or excessive mental stress, which may result from excessive worrying, lack of spiritual direction, among other factors. For successful treatment such adverse conditions must be eliminated. After all, what is the use of giving a person medicine if he insists on poisoning his system? If these conditions are met, I have no doubt that the germanium compound will cure the majority of cases of diseases which heretofore have been classified as showing poor response to medical treatment. Considering the nature of the substance—one which heals by instituting a condition of health throughout the whole body, (as opposed to substances which are used in specific treatments) every effort must be made to give full play to the body's own healing powers.

Jules Henri Poincaré has said that truth was no more than a hypothesis by which the greatest number of facts were explained under the simplest principles and without contradictions. My organic germanium compound has proved effective against all sorts of diseases, including cancers of the lung, bladder, larynx and breast, neurosis, asthma, diabetes, hypertension, cardiac insufficiency, inflammation of maxillary sinus, neuralgia, leukemia, softening of the brain, myoma of the uterus and hepatic cirrhosis. If a line that runs through the many cases of cure taken as isolated points should be found and an hypothesis known to be true should be set up, I should say that all diseases are attributable to deficiency of oxygen. The dangers of an oxygen deficiency in the human body cannot be overemphasized. I am not particularly trying to take a leaf out of a wise man's book by saying that "a balanced diet is an iron rule for staying healthy." This has been the cardinal principle of Oriental medicine and has been well recognized by modern Western medicine.

Germanium greatly enriches oxygen in the living body. Everyone knows that oxygen is absolutely essential for sustaining life, and there is no denying that all diseases are attributable to deficiency of oxygen in the body. Be it cancer, heart disease or mental disease, each undeniably strikes when oxygen deficiency within the body occurs. It is known that consumption of oxygen in the air has increased terrifyingly with the progress made in modern civilization. There is, in fact, an incident about a scientist, who blanched with fear when he found, by desk-top calculations, that oxygen in the air will be reduced by 0.8 per cent in fifteen years and that collective deaths of people will take place. This is no laughing matter; neither is the vogue of predicting possible extinction of mankind in fifteen to twenty years.

I have confirmed with my own body that my organic germanium compound not only radically enriches oxygen in the body but also expels pernicious pollutants from the body or at least decomposes them into harmless substances.

In the pages that follow I shall attempt to reveal the nature and wonder of organic germanium in relation to men's hearts, minds, and bodies.

Biological Significance of Germanium

1. The Element Germanium: Historical Background

Since its discovery, the history of germanium (atomic number 32, atomic weight 72.60, density 5.36) has been full of interesting episodes. The existence of the germanium element was foreseen about 100 years ago by the Russian chemist, Dmitri Mendeleev. Mendeleev, the proponent of the periodic law*, not only listed the properties of the then known elements but also theorized the existence of several undiscovered elements. In his periodic table, which he used to illustrate the law, he left certain gaps for the yet to be discovered elements—the 32nd column was for an element whose properties he predicted referred to as "ekasilicon." Mendeleev's theory of new elements proved correct. They began to appear with qualities remarkably similar to those which he predicted: Two appeared soon after he announced the law—gallium in 1875 and scandium in 1879.

In 1886, a German chemist, Clemens Winkler, while making a chemical analysis of the ore argyrodite, noticed on completion of his analysis that the sum of all the ingredients did not add up to the original quantity. At first he attributed this to some substance that escaped in the vapor produced with the ore which was being heated with chlorine ions in an acid solution. In efforts to locate the missing substance, he developed and experimented with several assays until he eventually succeeded in isolating it. In subsequent analyses he discovered that it fitted the description of the element Mendeleev

---

*A chemical law which states that the properties of the elements are periodic functions of their atomic weights.

had earlier called "ekasilicon." Winkler decided to name the new element germanium, in tribute to his fatherland.

2. Germanium: A Semiconductor

For the next 60 years germanium received little attention, remaining a subject of scientific study merely as a rare element. In 1948, however, it came to be utilized for its semiconducting characteristics by Brattain, Bardeen, and Shockley of the U.S. Bell Telephone Laboratories in the development of transistors and diodes, both of which came to play a leading role in modern electronics—transistors by replacing vacuum tubes as amplifiers, and diodes by becoming excellent rectifiers.

With the advent of these solid-state devices, germanium came to play a major role in the development of modern civilization from within the field of electronics. With worldwide attention centered on the characteristics of germanium as a semiconductor, its potential role in the field of biochemistry went virtually unnoticed. Research conducted on its possible applications in other fields brought few results and gained little momentum.

In appearance germanium is a metal, but it is completely without metallic properties. Many scientists in various countries refer to it as a nonmetal, while in Japan we tend to classify it as a semimetal. Usually, it is referred to merely as a semiconducting substance. In the classical school of physics, the characteristics of semiconductors were not clearly defined, and an adequate explanation for them was not given until the advent of quantum physics which is centered on the phenomena of effects produced by atomic and molecular electrons. Electronics engineers have since come to marvel at the whimsical and magic-like behavior of semiconductor electrons, and the quantum revolution soon spread to other fields. In the field of biochemistry, quantum biology and electrobiology emerged.

Whilst reading about these new fields of science, the thought of the characteristics of germanium, always in the back of my mind, flashed before me. Germanium electrons had been known to exhibit an uncommon behavior and I started thinking.

Germanium, atomic number 32, has 32 electrons, four of which are constantly moving unsteadily along the outermost shell of the atom. These four electrons are negative electrical charge carriers and if approached by a foreign substance one will be ejected out of its orbit. This famous phenomenon is known in electronics as the positive-hole effect which is so ingeniously utilized in forming transistors and diodes. When one of these four electrons is ejected, a positive-charge hole is created and the remaining three seize electrons from other atoms in order to maintain balance.

The thought came to me almost intuitively, but one day when I was dwelling on the fact that living organisms also come under the physical laws of matter, I was led to make a hypothetical supposition as to the effects that the semiconductor phenomenon would have on a living body.

Since there exists in physiology a phenomenon known as the dehydrogenating effect by which the negative ion of hydrogen (which may be viewed as an electron) is discharged from the body, I was led to the assumption that germanium might have interesting biological applications as well.*

3. The Existence of Germanium in Coal

My discovery of the biochemical significance of germanium occurred as follows. Towards the end of 1945 I was granted a permit to establish the Coal Research Center Foundation. My young researchers and I were motivated by the belief that the rebuilding of Japan's industries after the war depended on coal. Since we were working in the public interest naturally we felt that we should operate as a non-profit foundation. This research center provided the

---

*Dr. Asai discusses the relationship of living organisms and physics in a subsequent section, "Man—An Aggregate of Ultra Microscopic Electricity." The concept of dehydrogenation will also become apparent in subsequent sections. Briefly stated, it refers to the action of organic germanium in seizing and combining with hydrogen ions which have accumulated in the body to remove them.

womb that gave birth to my organic germanium. Conditions at the time were very confused, and even if there had been money there could be no research. Not only then but over many years there were periods of great hardship and it was only through great self-sacrifice on the part of myself, my family and loyal colleagues that the organic germanium compound came into existence.

I had gained the knowledge that coal contains germanium from Russian literature on the subject. Furthermore, when I was called to serve as an interpreter in the Scientific Resources Bureau set up by the American occupation forces I chanced to hear an American officer tell how there was a report on the rare element germanium in a document confiscated in Germany (the *PB report*) and how it declared this element would rule the future. There is still some doubt as to whether this was contained in the *PB report*, but it did serve to create an interest in the subject. An opportunity had opened up, and the fact that such an interest developed leads one to wonder whether or not it was after all an inevitability rather than mere chance. Or, may not the fact that this led to an unusual interest in the element germanium be the action of a dimension far above the ordinary?

At once, I had the staff investigate the amount of germanium to be found in coal. The microanalysis of a rare element demands superior knowledge and precision instruments. The staff and I worked unsparingly for nearly a year to establish a quantitative analysis of germanium. As we did not have funds to acquire the necessary instruments, we utilized those of other research centers.

Right after the war, about the only amusement was the movies and at that time the film "Madam Curie" was being shown, and I took the time to see it. Even today I cannot forget the excitement I felt at the end of that film. It was the impressive story of how Madam Curie with a crude store room for a laboratory, and with kettles, buckets, tubs, and the like, had succeeded in separating radium from pitchblende, and with the radium she had extracted, produced a strange light on a fluorescent screen. The film was pure inspiration. My staff also saw it and I pointed out to them that research involved more than material things; it demands much in the spiritual realm.

Coal is formed from the remains of ancient vegetation carbonized in an air-tight state as a result of complete immersion in seawater when swamp lands subsided millions of years ago. In coal petrography, a black lump of coal is classified and measured in three sections for the purposes of quantitative analyses: (1) Vitrit: the basically woody tissue, (2) Clarit: a hardened mixture of bark, leaves and twigs, and (3) Durit: a hardened mass of seeds and spores.

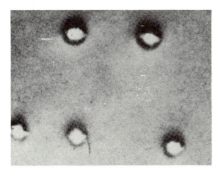

Vitrit
The basically woody tissue.

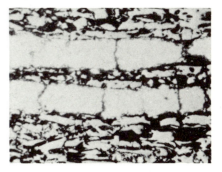

Clarit
A hardened mixture of bark, leaves and twigs.

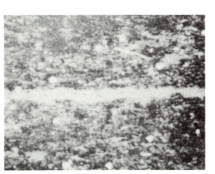

Durit
A hardened mass of seeds and spores.

It became clear that germanium was to be found in Japanese coal, about 5 to 10 parts per million (ppm). I learned that germanium is especially abundant in the vitrit or woody section. It occurs in comparatively small quantities in the older coals of the Coal Age—mainly the European and American varieties, of which the original plants were of the fern family—while coals of the younger Tertiary Period, such as those formed principally of the Sequois-dendron giganteum (a tree of the redwood family) commonly found in Japan and East Asia, contain a considerable amount of germanium.

4. Germanium and Plants

During the course of my analysis, I became curious as to why the wood section of the coal contained such particularly large quantities of germanium. On further examination of various coals, I detected the existence of medullary tubes, which are the vessels that plants use to draw nutrients from the soil. In short, I reasoned, the germanium in coal was first of all in the plants which were the source of the coal. In other words, it was primarily in living matter, and in my judgment, did not enter the coal later from the surrounding soil or mud.

New discoveries engender doubts and opposing views. As might be expected, the scholarly experts violently ridiculed my theory. For my part, however, the connection between germanium and plant life was too clear to be doubted. I saw a definite need to further clarify the relationship between plants and germanium. I turned to an acquaintance of mine in the Ministry of Agriculture and Forestry who assisted me in obtaining nearly 40 varieties of different species of bamboo from various parts of the country. I conducted a microanalysis of each of the samples and, as such advanced analytical equipment as an atomic absorption photometer was not available in those days, the time involved in this work was incredibly long. My efforts were fruitful, however. Analysis showed that several varieties of bamboo grass contained 15 to 20 ppm of germanium. This is a significant amount in the light of the critical amounts of such pollutants as small as one ppm of organic mercury in foodstuff or one ppm of sulfurous acid in the atmosphere considered fatal to living things. Viewed from this perspective I could not help thinking that the particularly large amounts of germanium in the bamboo grass must be of importance to its existence.

Continuing my analysis with other plants, I detected considerable amounts of germanium in tea leaves, oak leaves, chlorella, and so forth. I soon began to suspect that the existence of germanium in these plants has some connection with chlorophyll, with germanium perhaps acting as a catalyst with chlorophyll. Again, to consider the semiconductor characteristics of germanium, there is also the recently discovered Honda-Fujishima effect whereby a semiconductor placed in water and exposed to sunlight acts as a photo-electrochemical cell electrolyzing water into oxygen and hydrogen.* In terms of plant biology, when water is broken down into oxygen and hydrogen by this method, oxygen is discharged from the plant and hydrogen combines with the carbon of carbon dioxide absorbed by the plant to form carbohydrate. In effect, this means that in the process of assimilation plants produce starch sugar electrochemically from water only, a fact which seems to verify that germanium or some other semiconducting substance is essential to the growth of plants. In fact, although in quantities which vary a great deal from plant to plant, all plants seem to contain germanium. Observing such phenomena, I was astonished at how the laws of nature seemed to support the hypothesis that germanium plays a very important role in relation to biochemical life. Discoveries lending verification, however, followed in rapid succession.

I was further surprised to find that the plants containing unusually large quantities of germanium were without exception those valued as Chinese medicinal herbs. This discovery renewed my admiration for the accumulated wisdom and experience of Oriental medicine with its 2,000-year history, and added to my incentive to uncover the biochemical effects of germanium. My first steps were to measure the germanium content of those plants reputed to have beneficial

---

*"Electrochemical photolysis of Water at a Semiconductor Electrode" *Nature*. Vol. 238, July 7, 1972, 37.

effects in the treatment of malignant tumors. I obtained the following results.

Shelf fungus (*Trametes cinnabarina Fr.*)	800–2000 ppm
Ginseng (from Shimane Prefecture, Japan)	250 ppm
Ginseng (from Shinano district, Japan)	320 ppm
Sanzukon (*Codonopsis Tangshen*)	257 ppm
Sushi (*Angelica pubescens Maxim.*)	262 ppm
Waternut (*Trapa japonica Flerov*)	239 ppm
Boxthorn seed (*Lycium Chinese mill*)	124 ppm
Wisteria knob (gall) (*Wisteria floribunda*)	108 ppm
Pearl barley (*Coicis Semen*)	50 ppm
Gromwell (*Lithosemi Radix*) (*Lithospermum officinale*)	88 ppm

Shelf fungus, heading the list above, for centuries has been reputed to be effective in the treatment of cancer, and Nobel Prize winner Alexander Solzhenitsyn has even referred to this remarkable herb in his book, *Cancer Ward*.

Another plant reported to be effective in the treatment of cancer is a moss found in a small area of the Japanese countryside. I obtained some and was moved rather strangely to find that it also contained a rather large amount (250 ppm) of germanium. It should be pointed out, however, as later research revealed, 250 ppm is far from being an effective dosage against cancer.

Next, I analyzed those plants which are generally regarded as conducive to good health and found that they also contain fairly large quantities of germanium:

Aloe	77 ppm
Comfrey (*Symphytum Peregimum*)	152 ppm
Chlorella	76 ppm
Garlic	754 ppm
Bandai udo (*Aralia cordata*)	72 ppm
Bandai moss	255 ppm

Note: The germanium content of the plants analyzed in both of the above lists is not distributed evenly throughout the plant body. With ginseng, for example, even ginseng grown in Chinshan, Korea, where the world's most fertile crops of ginseng are produced, germanium is concentrated in the area extending from the center of the roots to the stems of the leaves; while the heavily concentrated area registers as much as 4,000 ppm, the peripheral root hairs contain no germanium at all.

Results of the above analyses and subsequent experiments eventually enabled me to give a plausible explanation for the presence of germanium in plants. Ginseng, for example, will not grow freely but requires soil of a particular consistency. Even then, from ancient times it has been known that after one good crop it takes up to 30 years to produce another crop of harvestable quality in the same soil. I conducted an experiment by obtaining ginseng sprouts approximately 8 cm in length and planted them in separate boxes. One box was sprinkled with a solution of germanium acetate and the other was left untreated. Six months later, the sprouts to which the germanium acetate was given had grown to a height of 30 cm and gave off the distinct aroma of ginseng. In contrast, the sprouts in the second box had grown to about 10 cm and gave off only a faint scent of ginseng. Obviously, germanium played an important role in the growth of this plant.*

5. A Weapon for Self-defense

For a more exact clue to the role germanium plays in plant life, it is interesting to note the wisteria plant. When attacked by germs and viruses, wisteria forms a knob (mentioned in the first list as containing a high concentration of germanium) in self-defense. This is a

---

*Ginseng is the common term for either of two herbs from the family Araliaceas, *Panax quinquefolium* and *Panax schinseng*. The former is the North American ginseng while the latter is common to Northeast Asia. Noted for its soothing properties, from time immemorial the Chinese have considered ginseng a cure for most illnesses, and the generic term "Panax" itself originates from a Greek word meaning "Panacea."

strong indication that the plant is using germanium to fight off the invading viruses. Further evidence that germanium serves to combat viruses in plants is a species of bamboo grass common to Yakushima* which received wide notice a number of years ago for its effectiveness in treating cancer. I obtained some and confirmed the presence of germanium in this plant. After a number of people had plucked the leaves, however, the roots began to weaken. What became apparent, in line with my theories was that the plant's ability to resist bacteria was lowered due to a disruption of the germanium cycle. The germanium existing in the soil, which is normally absorbed by the roots and returned to the soil when the leaves die and fall, was no longer present in adequate supply. Consequently, the plant became defenseless against bacteria and decayed. The same theory holds for ginseng also, which would be just as susceptible to the thousands of viruses and bacteria existing in the soil and would soon rot if it were not for its extremely high germanium content. One reason why, until recently, it has taken so long to cultivate regular crops of ginseng is that when one crop is harvested the germanium content is removed from the soil. A recent report says that success has been attained in harvesting an annual crop of ginseng by thoroughly disinfecting the soil. Although the beneficial effects of ginseng grown without germanium may be rather dubious, I believe the report re-emphasizes the role of germanium.

In addition to the plants mentioned above, germanium is also present in the structure of various mushrooms such as Cortinellus shiitake, champignon, and kawaradake. All these mushrooms are susceptible to various diseases and could not exist without sufficient resistance to bacteria. Interested in finding out more about the antibiotic properties of germanium, I conducted the following two experiments.

Experiment 1. A gelatine commonly used for the cultivation of bacteria was stained with methylene blue and put into five test tubes. Ten varieties of bacteria were then introduced into the gela-

---

*An island located in the southern part of Kyushu, Japan.

tine at random and a solution of germanium complex salt was poured into two of the five tubes. Since various bacteria require oxygen from the methylene blue to propagate themselves, the methylene blue takes on a transparent grey after the oxygen has been used. In the tubes containing germanium, however, the methylene blue maintained its original color, indicating that the bacteria died, being unable to utilize the oxygen.

Experiment 2. Using another method for cultivating bacteria, gelatine was put on two test plates—one containing germanium and one without it. Various microorganisms were introduced and molds of various colors began to grow on the surface of the gelatine without germanium. No change occurred, however, on the plate containing germanium.

However, about a week later, dark spots appeared on the surface of the test plates of gelatine containing germanium used in Experiment 2. In no time the spots, appearing to be miniature aegagropilas in form and color, developed into well-rounded spheres about 7mm in diameter. Nonetheless, when viewed from a different angle, the above phenomenon, rather than indicating failure, merely re-emphasized the effectiveness of the germanium solution. The bacteria used in the first experiment died because their molecular structure was destroyed by the dehydrogenating effect, or oxidizing action of germanium. The mold which grew on the test plate containing germanium used in Experiment 2, however, grew principally due to the presence of germanium—a large mold resembling aegagropilas could not have grown without germanium because the microorganisms present would have destroyed it before it was established. The mold made use of the germanium to fight harmful bacteria as well as to facilitate its own growth.

In an experiment with rice plants I discovered another effect of germanium: it increases their resistance to cold. In a greenhouse, rice was grown at a temperature of about 20°C having first been immersed in a germanium solution for two days. When the rice grew to a height of about 30cm, the temperature of the greenhouse was

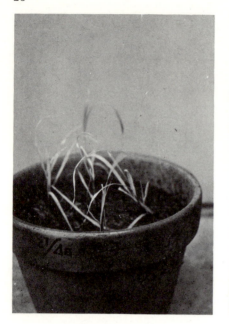
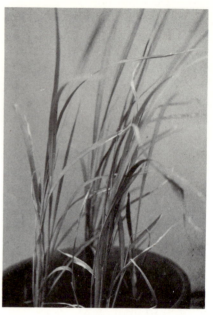

Rice plants
not given germanium (5°C)

Rice plants
given germanium (5°C)

lowered to 5°C. As a result, the rice plants grown from the unhulled rice which had not been immersed in the germanium solution soon withered and rotted from the cold. The plants grown from the unhulled rice treated with germanium, however, were unharmed by the cold and steadily continued their healthy growth.

Various other experiments led to the observation of other interesting phenomena. When only a small quantity of the germanium solution was used, the growth of various plants was greatly accelerated and their flowering period was advanced. Germanium was also found to have positive effects on plant cuttings. Improved assimilation was noted when water drawn by the plants was electrolyzed by sunlight with germanium acting as a catalyst.

All these experiments pointed to a very interesting relationship existing between living substances and metals. In nature there is a transmigrational phenomenon whereby metallic elements existing in the soil play an important part in plant growth when absorbed by plants. Animals absorb these elements after feeding on the plants and return them to the soil through evacuation or upon death. Naturally, the metallic elements involved in this cycle move in organic form from the plant to animal bodies, and I became extremely interested in determining what form of organic compound is present in living organisms. If this organic compound could be found and synthesized, a substance could be created which would surely have beneficial effects on all forms of life.

The physicist Schrodinger said, "Life is a supreme work of art created by the hands of God through quantum mechanics." Since I was setting out to create a substance of vital importance to life which this great scientist referred to as God's work of art, I had to adopt the proper frame of mind. The physical laws of nature are complicated so that the creation of a new substance is the most difficult of problems. To this end, in a spirit of prayer to God, I have undergone extreme hardship and devoted thirty years of my life.

6. Synthesis of Organic Germanium Compound

To invent is not the conquest of nature. Man creates nothing, he merely uncovers things which were heretofore unknown.

The synthesis of organic germanium has fulfilled a vision I have had since youth of doing something good for mankind. However, it was not an easy task. Research on the organic germanium compound progressed smoothly at first. Working with germanium in organic form was not entirely new to me for I had previously met with considerable success by extracting germanium from coal in the early 1950's. I had also succeeded in obtaining large quantities from liquefied coal gas. Previous research activities had been directed primarily at obtaining an inorganic germanium of a high purity for use by the electronics industry.

To extract germanium from coal, I developed a process whereby the organic germanium in coal is removed at high temperature in a carbonization furnace. It is then liquefied by adjusting the pH and burned to eliminate miscellaneous organics. Afterwards, it is chlori-

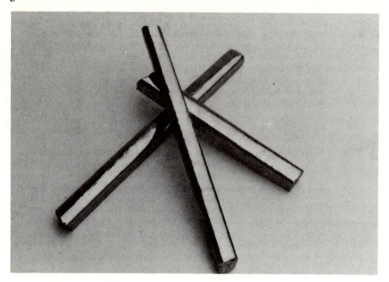

The single crystal of germanium

nated and this chlorinated organic germanium is converted by hydrolysis into germanium oxide, a white powder, further reduced by hydrogen. Increased purity is achieved by zone melting, and finally a lump of cylindrical-shaped silver-gray single crystals is produced.

The principal object of my research with germanium until that point had been to convert the organic germanium obtained from coal into an inorganic substance for the electronics industry.

I was now faced with doing the reverse in converting inorganic germanium into an organic substance if it was to be of use in the field of biochemistry. I first thought that in order to obtain a germanium compound which is biochemically active, the synthetic germanium must be made with an affinity to living cells. My research staff and I studied the possibility of compounding germanium with either amino acid or nucleic acid. We attacked these and other possibilities from every angle, but our attempts failed. At the time, publications on germanium in Japanese or any other language were virtually nonexistent and ten years went by almost completely unnoticed while we were groping in the dark. In the meantime, the once flourishing coal industry had reached its zenith and began to decline from around 1959. With the decline, the royalties and research grants which I had been receiving from coal mining companies for my discoveries decreased sharply. My personal finances were also nearly exhausted, and it became increasingly difficult to run a research laboratory. I often say, "Poverty and affliction are the mother of invention." Once I discussed this matter with Dr. Reppe, a German scientist who had been awarded the Nobel prize for his work in the chemistry of acetylene. He said, "Invention is made up of 90% perspiration and 10% gray matter."

Whilst trying to combat and resolve these difficulties I realized the danger of losing my creative spirit. I began to read fervently *From Religion to Science* by Bertrand Russell; *Einstein and the Order of Space; Zen and the Art of Archery* by Eugen Herrigel; *Dogen* (about a Zen work), and several other books by Japanese authors. I made notes of the thoughts of great men and these supplied the thread that kept me from succumbing completely. The saying which sticks uppermost in mind, however, is—"God may give you a chestnut but won't crack it and take it out of the shell for you."

In November, 1967, a member of my research staff who stayed on, walked into the room holding a test tube of white powder. Raising it slowly, and with an expression on his face which radiated the whole room, he uttered the words I had been waiting ten years to hear: "Dr. Asai, the water-soluble organic germanium compound has at last been synthesized." For the first time in my life I shed tears of joy in deep silence as a man in ecstacy. They were tears of almost religious exaltation. The event proved to me that all of man's struggles are not in vain. The organic germanium compound synthesized on that day has changed my life, and as I hope you shall see, has done something good for everyone who has come in contact with it.

7. Myself as the Living Body Test

The newly synthesized water-soluble germanium compound has been a blessing in every sense of the word. Technically termed carboxy ethyl sesquioxide of germanium (GeCH$_2$CH$_2$COOH)$_2$O$_2$* it features three oxygen atoms affixed to each germanium atom as indicated in the figure below. Germanium has four electrons available for shar-

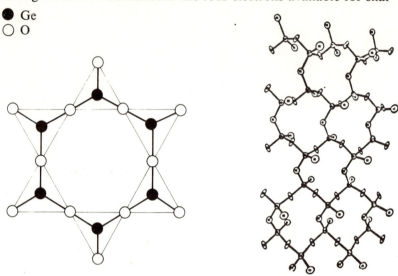

A beautiful geometrical pattern seen in the reticular structure of germanium

ing: one is a free radical (not shown in the figure), while the other three are affixed alternately to an oxygen atom. The oxygen atoms, in turn, combine with germanium atoms in a manner resembling a bed of flowers or a regularly expanding gymnastic formation. Each time I view this substance which so magnificently illustrates the laws of nature and contains the potential to alter the course of life, Einstein's words "The perception of mystery is the source of every learning and discovery," come to mind.

Till the discovery of the compound, I had managed to keep myself in fairly good spirits by reading, but my physical condition had deteriorated, and I was in a state of virtual disability. Doctors had diagnosed my illness as a severe case of polyrheumatism complicated

---

*Refer to Appendix 1 The Organo Germanium Sesquioxide.

by arthritis and had given little hope of improvement. True, the organic germanium compound had just been synthesized, but it was still in the experimental stage. Usually with a new medicine, extensive toxicity tests are made before it is used on people. I decided that my own illness would be its first real test. My decision was not entirely based on blind faith, however. Prior to the discovery, my years of research with plants and animals had indicated that its overall effect would be beneficial, or harmless at least. Furthermore, some scientific data from the Soviet Union indicated that germanium was nontoxic.

I took some of the white, powdery organic germanium with water. Improvement was slow at first, but I continued to take the solution in large dosages for several days. Gradually, I began to feel better and in ten days I was up and walking around the house—at times feeling robustly healthy.

Since the rheumatic affliction I was suffering from is generally regarded as incurable by modern medicine, I had been visiting an acupuncturist in the neighborhood in an attempt to relieve my pains. Upon examination after only a few visits, the acupuncturist was astounded to find that my body had already healed to an unbelievable extent. Moreover, on a subsequent visit he requested some of the compound for his other patients, convinced that it would help them.

After taking it for several more weeks until I was assured that it was completely nontoxic, and that there was no sign of its accumulation in my body, however, I gave him some. Again, he was astounded as patients who had been suffering from a variety of diseases, heretofore regarded as virtually incurable—cancer, epilepsy, cirrhosis of the liver and a list of others—all showed marked improvement when administered the compound. Developments were indeed encouraging. Unfortunately, however, the acupuncturist was forced to discontinue treatment with germanium because it was pointed out to him that the use of germanium at this stage constituted an act against laws governing the use of medicine in Japan.

8. Effects on Animals

Before describing its effects in the human body I will mention a few examples of my germanium compound used in animals. It seems to have an almost miraculous efficacy in these cases. A Siamese cat at our home had been in the fangs of a dog during a wild fight. The wounds were so serious, we began fearing for its life. We started applying dressings to the wounds with a water solution of the organic germanium, at the same time forcing him to drink this solution. This was done in the presence of the veterinarian we had called. On calling again a few days later, he was almost dumbfounded at the rapid recovery of the cat, saying that he could now believe in miracles.

The large Japanese carp specially bred for decorative purposes, being artificially raised, are liable to contract diseases easily. An acquaintance who was keeping such carp reported to me that several had contracted a disease. Some of their scales were peeling off. Lying on their sides, they were gasping for air apparently on the verge of death. On my advice he put a pinch of the organic germanium compound into the water in which they were swimming, and to his utmost delight the fish soon began swimming vigorously, biting greedily at the feed in which they had showed no interest only a short while previously. The owner of the carp now claims that the organic germanium compound is indispensable for breeding carp.

Germanium showed the same curative effects on cats, dogs and horses where diseases withstood treatment in the conventional manner, so that many veterinarians have strongly requested that the organic germanium compound be made available for general use as soon as possible. Bird lovers who used germanium on their ailing birds have also expressed their delight at its efficacy.

A female Dobermann imported from England was mated seven times within 5 years but did not conceive once. The owner became worried that the dog would age without giving him a litter. As a last resort he turned to intravenous and subcutaneous injections of organic germanium one month before the dog came into heat. These injections were continued all through the mating season. This time the dog conceived, delivering a litter of five males and six females, all healthy puppies, mother and children doing well to the utmost delight of their owner.

No matter how much is given to animals, there is no lethal level to report. The more they get, the more active they become. In the Drugs, Cosmetics, and Medical Instruments Act, the lethal amount is reached if half the animals die. With germanium there is no lethal amount. Therefore, it is not a medicine.

9. Germanium as an Experimental Medicine

Having virtually recovered from my own disease, and witnessed the mysterious healing action of the organic germanium compound, I became anxious to see it put to use for medical treatment. I wasted no time in initiating toxicity tests with animals at an authoritative research institute. The tests they ran included those for acute, subacute, and chronic toxicity, as well as deformity-producing effects. The results of all the tests showed the compound to be completely nontoxic and harmless. (Refer to Appendix 2-1, 2-2, Toxicity of Organo Germanium.)

With thorough assurance that the compound was nontoxic, I was able to obtain financial backing and opened a clinic on the outskirts of Tokyo. My doctor friends agreed to rely on germanium as much as possible in their treatment, and together we witnessed the remarkable recovery of patients with diseases that had hardly responded to medical treatment. Thorough records of the patients' reactions to treatment and course of recovery were maintained to develop an adequate explanation of the mechanism by which the compound heals.

People taking my organic germanium continued to do so in increasing numbers when they saw its remarkable results. I gave it to them at cost, just enough for research expense, and laid down the following two provisions: First of all, my organic germanium should never be considered a medicine. It enriches the body's oxygen supply, and one is cured from disease by his own powers. One must put great trust in germanium, and pay close attention to his diet in order to avoid constitutional acidity. Secondly, I have labored earnestly for more than 20 years, motivated always by a vision that the organic germanium I was producing was a godsend from heaven to alleviate human suffering and to save humanity from disease. That means that the sick must take only germanium, add prayer to it and use no medicine in addition. If used in conjunction with other medicines its effectiveness is diminished.

The great surgeon and scientist, Alexis Carrel, has said:

"Although man has been fascinated by the remarkable progress that science has made in dealing with unliving things and inanimate objects, he has as yet failed to realize that the flesh and minds of human beings are also governed by laws which are as precise as the world of stars and many times as mysterious. Moreover, he is ignorant of the danger inherent in the violation of such laws." (Alexis Carrel: *Man, the Unknown*)

Watching the effect of the compound on the patients at our clinic, these words came to mind. It seemed as if germanium were a substance springing from a yet unknown dimension with a direct link to the vital forces of life.

I am a scientist, however, and well aware of the dangers of non-empirical thinking and soon set about to define the mechanism of the compound in scientific terms. By watching all the changes that took place with patients following the administration of the compound, I was able to conclude that its healing powers may be attributed to the fact that it brings about a sharp increase in the body's supply of oxygen: A patient will feel a certain warmth surging throughout his body within 10 minutes or so after taking the compound—some people actually feel as if they have been given a mixture that included alcohol. Yawning soon ceases, blood becomes less viscous and complexions take on a healthy glow. Carbon monoxide poisoning is quickly cured, and people feel cheerful, sleep soundly and wake in good humor. They also show evidence of increased mental powers, along with numerous other overall positive effects which will be described in more detail in later sections.

10. Mechanism of Action

Morbid tissues are generally characterized by oxygen deficiency. Accumulation of H^+ radicals tends to destroy cells and tissues which gradually accumulate to cause disorders which in turn deteriorate in a morbid condition generated for various reasons. If oxygen could be selectively and locally fed to this lesion, oxygen would combine with the accumulated H^+ radicals to restore the deteriorated tissues, thereby cutting the vicious circle of accumulation of deteriorated tissues and disorders, restoring the normal functions of the tissues.

The basis of the theory of the mechanism of the compound is that germanium takes the form of a sesquioxide:

$$Ge\begin{matrix}\nearrow O-\\ -O-\\ \searrow O-\end{matrix}$$

Oxygen readily combines with hydrogen, so it becomes apparent that hydrogen will strongly bind with the oxygen atoms of the compound, consequently bringing about a dehydrogenating reaction which is the mechanism by which germanium eliminates harmful substances causing disease in the body.

Consider for a moment the basic fact of the life process whereby food is burned by the body to give energy, while carbon dioxide (CO_2) and hydrogen (H_2) are created. CO_2 is discharged from the lungs when we exhale, and H_2 combines with oxygen to form water which is discharged in the urine and sweat. As mentioned previously, hydrogen may be referred to as a positive ion, which is as useless to the body as dust clogging the workings of a machine.

To insure that the body functions normally, hydrogen must be removed, but for complete removal a large quantity of oxygen is needed. The germanium compound with its strong dehydrogenating effect takes the place of oxygen in combining with hydrogen to eliminate the latter from the body. In fact, all traces of germanium are discharged from the body through the digestive tract within 20 to 30 hours.

As part of another experiment, tests were conducted on the effect of the germanium compound on the respiratory tissues of a group of mice using the Warburg method. Results obtained showed a remarkable decrease of oxygen consumption in the diaphragm and liver—clear indication that the compound acted as a substitute for oxygen in combining with hydrogen. By the dehydrogenating or oxidizing action of the compound, not only hydrogen ions are removed from the blood, but abnormal proteins and other foreign matter are also removed. The oxidizing effect of the compound thus serves to purify the blood.

11. A Substitute for Oxygen

The organic germanium compound increases the oxygen supply in a living body. The compound leads to the cure of various diseases and produces health-sustaining effects by serving as a substitute for oxygen in combining with hydrogen ions and other waste substances in the body.

In the following experiment, for example, the germanium compound was given orally to a rat in amounts calculated at 30mg per kilogram of its body weight. When the rat was examined 1 $1/2$ hrs later, the distribution of germanium in its body was found to be as follows:

Distribution of Organic Germanium in Parts Per Million
(Male Wistar Rat 180g receiving 30mg/kg body weight)

lung	22.5 ppm
heart	2.5 ppm
stomach	188.0 ppm
liver	12.0 ppm
kidney	15.0 ppm
spleen	27.5 ppm
testicles	8.0 ppm
urine	90.0 ppm
small intestine	522.0 ppm
mucous membrane of small intestine	788.0 ppm
contents of small intestine	507.6 ppm

caecum and large intestine	10.5 ppm
mucous membrane of caecum and large intestine	8.0 ppm
contents of caecum and large intestine	15.5 ppm
cerebral bone	21.5 ppm
blood	43.2 ppm

As is shown in the table, only 1 $^1/_2$ hrs after administration, a large amount of the compound still remains in the stomach as it has not yet been absorbed. It is also evident, however, that the germanium content in the blood is still relatively high. In the blood, it is believed that germanium combines mostly with red blood cells—a theory which can be deduced from the fact that red blood cells, which are negative charge carriers and have properties permitting penetration by negative ions, have an electrochemical structure closely akin to the germanium compound. Thus, it appears that germanium combines with the red blood cells together with hemoglobin.

In the ensuing pages of this book I propose to develop the concept of my organic germanium compound as a health-giving substance rather than a medicine and through the weight of personal evidence provide a more complete way of life.

From the Logical World of Science to the Mystic World of God

1. Miracle Waters

The writings of Alexis Carrel have had a great influence on my concept of life. In 1912 he won the Nobel prize for physiology and medicine for his origination of the Carrel suture, a technique for suturing blood vessels, and for his work in transplanting internal organs. He was a true scientist but he recognized a world that transcends science. He believed in that world and that is what interested me most. His intimate friend, Dr. Lindbergh, an American physician and doctor of philosophy, wrote this, "Carrel's spirit as with the speed of light crosses from the world of logical science to the mystic world of God and back again."

Carrel says this, "We must be freed from the universe created by scientists with their marvelous intelligence. We stand in awe before the great expanse of the material world, but it is too narrow for mankind. I cannot believe that we are hedged in by the confines of this material world. We know that we have a wider expanse that transcends the physical."

Carrel's treatment of the phenomenon of crossing over the boundaries of science began as a result, it is said, of his visit to Lourdes. The sick who go to Lourdes drink the holy water, or those with serious illness bathe in it, and they declare they are healed. Carrel made careful observations of the large number of the sick who came every year and are saved by the "miracle water." This led him to a new concept of science and religion and to the discovery of a great

Germanium and Health

1. Well-Balanced Diet, Prerequisite to Good Health

As will be seen later, the organic germanium compound can be regarded without exaggeration as an effective means of combating almost any disease. Nonetheless, for assuring its efficacy and the health of the body, the following two conditions have to be met. One is to keep a well-balanced diet in order to maintain the acidalkali equilibrium of the body fluids. The other is to relieve stress to keep a stable mental state for maintaining the equilibrium of the autonomic nervous system. If any one of these equilibria is broken, a morbid change is likely to occur somewhere in the body.

The oxygen needed for the human body is supplied through respiration, and observing the necessities for the maintenance of human life, the first thought is the need for oxygen supplied to the body through respiration, while the need for nourishment in the form of water and food and sleep follow a close second. If oxygen supply to the brain is suspended for more than three minutes, the brain fails to recover consciousness. If water intake is suspended for about a week, dehydration causes death. If no sleep is obtained for a week, mental disorder caused by lack of sleep results in complete mental derangement. Only if the three foregoing conditions are met, can a healthy person go without food for one month.

With these conditions in mind, it is up to man to choose the proper type of food. For this reason, it is important to keep a well-balanced diet. For maintaining health or curing a disease, it is of utmost importance to adhere to a diet that includes food which will keep the pH of the body fluids slightly alkaline at 7.2 to 7.4.

To facilitate a judicious selection, the following classification points out types of food that are termed either as acid-or alkali-forming:

HIGHLY ACID FOODS:	egg yolk, cheese, sweets in which white sugar is used, dried bonito, oyster, and herring-roe.
MODERATELY ACID FOODS:	ham, bacon, horse meat, chicken, tuna, pork, white bread, beef, wheat, butter, and eel.
SLIGHTLY ACID FOODS:	rice, peanuts, octopus, clams, liver, fried bean curd, and beer.
SLIGHTLY ALKALINE FOODS:	red beans, onions, cabbage, Japanese radishes, apples, a kind of chinese cabbage, and bean-curd.
MODERATELY ALKALINE FOODS:	raisins, soybeans, cucumbers, carrots, tomatoes, spinach, banana, tangerines, pumpkins, strawberries, honeywort, white of egg, pickled plums, and lemon.
HIGHLY ALKALINE FOODS:	seaweed, grapes, tea, and wine.

Acid foods when absorbed into the body tend to acidify the blood, while alkaline foods reverse this tendency toward acidosis.

Lemon juice will turn the blue litmus paper red as a test for acidity reaction will show, but once it is absorbed into the body, it acts to turn the blood alkaline. Thus, lemon is classified as an alkaline food.

Aside from those who are still growing, people should avoid excessive intake of animal protein and fats. They would do better to take soybeans and processed foods thereof, as well as vegetables. Vegetable fats are also better than animal fats. If people maintain a well-balanced diet centered on natural vegetable foods, they will be able to sustain good health since these increase resistance against diseases and reinforce natural curing ability should they fall victim to some ailment. Any diet partial to acid foods like meat and fatty fish meat, especially to animal foods, is tantamount to shortening one's life.

2. Pregnancy

The food 'fads' of pregnant women are of interest. My daughters began no longer to care for fatty foodstuffs or meats, while definitely preferring vegetables, fruit and pickled *ume* (a Japanese fruit similar to apricot and plum). All these foods are in the alkali group of foods.

In traditional Chinese medicine, acid and salt are described as the negative and the positive, respectively. The Chinese principle calls for maintaining equilibrium of the positive and the negative in diet. Chinese medicine classifies *umeboshi* in the negative, that is, the alkali group of foods. As I mentioned earlier, I was struck by the Chinese wisdom that listed pickled plums as a negative food despite its acidity which tends to mislead people to think of them as an acid-forming food.

This change of pattern in diet during pregnancy conforms to the need of the foetus in the womb of the mother. Oxygen is the most important substance for the growth of the foetus. If the mother has acidosis, there is sure to be oxygen deficiency which will adversely affect the foetus. I find a special providence in the natural change in the pattern of likes and dislikes in the diet of women in pregnancy.

The oriental antenatal training of expectant mothers in this connection should be interpreted in the light of the need for stabilizing their mental state, which keeps a well-balanced physical condition. My daughters took organic germanium daily during their pregnancy to maintain abundant oxygen supply to the body. Consequently, they experienced only very slight morning-sickness during the first few months of pregnancy and gave birth to strong, healthy babies in easy deliveries. Thus, I am endowed with six healthy grandchildren. Many similar cases are found in letters of appreciation I have received.

In one case, an expectant mother was diagnosed as having leukemia and had been advised by her doctor to arrange for an abortion. As she turned to germanium therapy which had an excellent effect on her leukemia, she was able to give birth to a fine boy. This is only one of many examples of the beneficial effect of germanium therapy in pregnancy.

Invariably they have an easy delivery and their babies are healthy and vigorous. I am sure the tragedy of giving birth to defective infants could be avoided if all pregnant women would take organic germanium.

3. Birth of Healthy Life

Here is a case reported in the newspapers. Parents of a premature baby, who lost its eyesight because of a retinal disorder whilst in an incubator, brought a lawsuit against the hospital for the damage caused to the child, only to lose the case. Prevention of retinal disorders in premature babies appears to be possible by applying the latest technology, but it seems that cases of this nature are not yet recognized as being attributable to hospital error.

Medical journals report an increasing number of premature births. That the health of prospective mothers is markedly deteriorating is undeniable when aggravation of environmental conditions due to food and pollution is taken into account. Imperfect physical conditions of prospective mothers are probably leading to an increased number of premature births.

In support of this statement, I would like to point out that pregnant women taking organic germanium all have smooth deliveries and that not one premature or physically-handicapped baby has been born to such a mother.

The reason is very simple. Germanium enriches the body with oxygen, and as the mother's womb remains in a wonderfully healthy condition, the fetus grows unimpeded.

While more about this matter is presented in another chapter, I would like to introduce the summary of a report submitted by Dr. Mieko Okazawa who is a member of the Infant Protection Association. Report submitted October 15, 1977.

Eight examples of perfectly healthy babies born to women taking organic germanium during pregnancy

Child's name	Weight and Height at Birth	Family relationship	Mother's age at time of delivery	Mother's condition
(1) H.Y. Dec. 24, 1974	Wt. 3,850g	Third child Eldest son	Born in 1946 28	
(2) T.K. Aug. 2, 1976	Wt. 3,175g	Second child Eldest son	Born in 1947 29	
(3) I.Y. Jan. 25, 1977	Wt. 4,130g Ht. 51cm	Fourth child Second son	Born in 1944 32 32	
(4) N.A. Jan. 31, 1977	Wt. 3,840g	Second child Second daughter	Born in 1950 26	
(5) S.T. May 28, 1977	Wt. 3,700g Ht. 53cm Bust 33cm Head 32cm	Second child Second son	Born in 1942 35	
(6) S.T. June 16, 1977	Wt. 3,580g Ht. 50.7cm Bust 34.5cm Head 34.5cm	Third child Third son	Born in 1943 33	
(7) S.A. Aug. 26, 1977	Wt. 3,950g Ht. 54cm	Second child Eldest daughter	Born in 1951 26	
(8) N.M. Oct. 5, 1977	Wt. 3,670g Ht. 49cm Bust 34cm	Second child Eldest daughter	Born in 1951 26	

Case 1. As both the eldest and the second daughter were sickly and the mother herself of weak constitution and as her urine was showing sugar (++) at the beginning of pregnancy, she began to take germanium (Ge) from the second month of pregnancy. She gave birth to a healthy boy. (She took 500cc Ge a month.)

Case 2. The woman began an intake of 200mg/day Ge because of a threatened abortion at 7 months. After her condition stabilized, the daily amount was reduced to 80mg.

Case 3. As all three of her children contracted German measles early in her fourth pregnancy, the mother began to take Ge. The intake was 80mg a day. In the eighth month of pregnancy she contracted influenza accompanied by coughing fits. She therefore was advised to increase the intake to 400mg to 500mg per day, later returning to 80mg a day till delivery.

Case 4. The woman suffered from toxemia of pregnancy and albumen in her urine while pregnant with her first child. When the second child was on the way, from the fifth month she began Ge intake until delivery which was smooth and she gave birth to a healthy baby.

Case 5. The woman was allergic to medication. She contracted influenza in the fourth month of pregnancy, accompanied by coughing fits. She began to take Ge only. As she suffered from coughing fits during the ninth month of pregnancy too, she was administered Ge injections in addition to oral Ge doses till delivery. She gave birth to a healthy baby.

Case 6. As the mother was in her mid-thirties by the time she conceived her third child, she began to take 100 mg of Ge per day from the initial period of pregnancy.

Case 7. The woman began to take 400 mg/day Ge from the ninth month of pregnancy because of albumen (0) in her urine, and dropsical swelling. While pregnant with her first child, she had fallen into pregnancy-phobia. She received a blood transfusion for profuse bleeding and experienced a difficult delivery; but this time she had an easy delivery probably as a result of taking Ge.

Case 8. The woman took Ge before her pregnancy on account of delicate health and autonomic ataxia. Serious vomiting, anemia during the latter part of pregnancy and a rise in blood pressure prompted her to have additional Ge injections while also orally taking Ge till delivery which went smoothly.

Note: Ge stands for organic Germanium.

I cannot help thinking that premature births and births of physically handicapped children result from some violation of the workings of nature. Nature fills the universe with rational equations and steadily flows with time. It should, therefore, be natural that perfectly normal babies be born. Yet, that this is not the case probably stems from the existence of something which is not in accord with the principles of nature.

That a life comes into this world is a profound mystery, originating from the time of conception and developing through the growth of the fetus over a long period. What is most needed during this period is oxygen obtained through the mother's respiration.

If the mother's blood is acid, the oxygen-carrying capacity of hemoglobin in the red blood cells markedly declines and this may lead to a failure to supply the interior of the womb with an adequate amount of oxygen. This creates a dangerous situation.

There are two causes of acidic blood. One is mental instability. The importance attached to the prospective mother's mental state since early days in the name of antenatal education is perfectly correct. The other cause is diet. Preferences for food change when a woman becomes pregnant, and dislike of acid-forming foods such as meat and fatty foods often develops. This is an admirable and marvelous example of the working of nature. Nature thus is doing her utmost to prevent a shortage of oxygen in the mother's womb, but if the womb becomes acidic through stress and polluted foodstuffs caused by the unhealthy habits of modern life, the child is liable to abort, be born prematurely or with physical defects.

It is, therefore, by no means an exaggeration to say that the use of germanium is absolutely necessary for a pregnant woman to assure the birth of a healthy child.

4. Reasons for Oxygen Deficit in the Body

Although I shall refer to the reason for ill-health together with the conditions for treatment of disease on many ocacsions, perhaps it would be useful to summarize the causes for an oxygen deficiency in the body at this point since this seems to be the root of all body disorders.

(i) Though acidity has long been recognized as a problem, perhaps one reason why ill-health is so rampant is that most people do not bother to find an adequate explanation as to why this condition is detrimental to health. Although it may sound complicated, the scientific answer is rather simple. An acid constitution means that the blood contains an excess of positive hydrogen ions (H^+) which use up the oxygen in a living body by combining with it to form an hydroxyl group. When an excess of (H^+) accumulates in the body, there is insufficient oxygen to consume them. As a consequence the blood will acidify and an oxygen deficiency will be created. The problem of oxygen deficiency has also become a controversy in recent years. An acid constitution should be averted by all means. An acid constitution leads to an oxygen deficiency which results in various diseases, including cancer.

(ii) The intake of foods which contain an excess of unsaturated chemical compounds can be noted as another major cause of oxygen deficiency. Unsaturated compounds have a surplus of molecular "hands" which combine with oxygen in the body to produce oxonium compounds, thereby depleting the body's supply of oxygen. In an experiment we conducted with dogs, one of the animals died from cancer induced by means of the above method. The chemical nature of substance is to move from an unsaturated state, at which they can establish their existence. In this context, it is important for those who want to stay healthy to note that natural foods contain the fewest unsaturated compounds, while these compounds are conspicuously abundant in refined foods. In my mind, carcinogenic or cancer-producing substances and unsaturated compounds—with their excess of molecular "hands" to use up the available oxygen in the body—are one and the same.

(iii) The other major cause of oxygen deficiency in the body, perhaps that to which we should pay the most attention, is the mind. A theory of Professor Hans Selye of the University of Montreal, Canada, is that not only humans but animals develop an unbalanced secretion of hormones, particularly adrenal hormones, if subjected to prolonged stress. An imbalanced hormone secretion will also lead to acidification of the blood and thereby create a condition for oxygen deficiency which ultimately results in disease. In an experiment we conducted in our laboratory, mice were encaged and poked with a stick to irritate and provoke them. Not surprisingly, upon dissection, it was found that all had developed stomach ulcers, some of which had hemorrhaged. An examination of their blood revealed the pH value had dropped by 0.2 on average, clearly indicating that the blood had become highly acidified.

With the recent remarkable progress in biochemistry, many warnings have been issued on the relationship between health and diet. Moreover, stress is fast becoming recognized as a major cause of disease. Again, I wish to re-emphasize the necessity of maintaining a constitution that will not produce an oxygen deficiency. This is a conclusion reached after several years of laboratory work with the organic germanium compound and, to date, all the facts have supported it without exception.

5. Stress

In order adequately to explain the interrelationship of germanium and health, particularly as regards the mind, it is necessary to draw together several fields of knowledge. By examination of some theories from the field of physics we may note that physics is a science dealing basically with the clarification of various phenomena which constitute the basis of matter. Human beings, by the very nature of the fact that they are composed of matter, are also governed by the theories of the properties of matter as expounded by physics. In terms of physics, as quantum theory has revealed, a human being is an aggregate of ultra-minute electrically-charged particles. You may wonder what all this has to do with disease. This does so precisely because the physical composition and behavior of matter is known to accord with the laws of nature. Although you may choose to agree or disagree with the hypothesis, scientific evidence has indicated it is important to man in terms of mental and physical health to have some basic direction in life.

Professor Selye maintains that disease develops from mental stress. Stress is "strain," and may be interpreted in terms of minute electrical particles which constitute the body. In effect, the occurrence of a disease means that one portion of the universe's equation has become incompatible with the rest.

The simplest way to detect stress (strain) is to measure the electrical potential of the various parts of the body. Each mass of electrical particles naturally has its own electrical potential. Brain troubles are diagnosed by brain waves. The principle involved in this type of examination is to locate the affected area of the brain by measuring the electrical potentials at various points. The same principle applies to the internal organs. There is an appropriate potential for the stomach, liver, heart, kidneys, pancreas and other organs. Once affected by disease, the potential of an organ, the source of which are the electrons, will either increase or fall. It is important to note that in the living body, the hydrogen ion, which is the source of an electrical potential, serves as this electron.

As an interesting side note on the relationship of germanium and electrical potentials, we conducted an experiment whereby a solution containing the organic germanium compound was poured into the battery of an automobile which had failed to start due to battery failure. The immediate result was that the car started without difficulty. Furthermore, batteries have been recharged without difficulty in a few minutes by adding a small quantity of the germanium compound. It is difficult to explain such phenomena scientifically, but it seems obvious that electrical potentials have been increased. The state of a human body, in which no electrical potentials may be detected, is death.

In recent years much more time has been devoted to the study of stress in connection with personality and profession. In this connection some interesting facts have come to light. First of all, the artist, working in an atmosphere of pure art apparently is not subject to undue stress. Their blood does not become acid, whereas the broker class seems always to be under irritation, worrying, and always in an uneasy state which results in blood acidity, an oxygen deficiency, and which finally ends in stomach ulcers. I have a friend who is head of the research laboratory in the National Police Agency. Once I inadvertently heard him say something that made me slap my knee and nod in agreement.

"When a criminal commits murder in connection with a robbery, he knows that if caught he faces execution, therefore he invariably looks for a chance to run away and hide. The police send notices to every city, town, and village office, but on the average, only about 60% of such culprits are caught. However, strangely enough, after four or five years, those not apprehended develop some incurable disease, very often cancer, and die. Along with the doctor's certificate of death, a report of the person's personal history is sent to the local office, and we know he is on the wanted list of criminals."

The criminal in hiding lives with fear and a guilty conscience day and night, and his body is under fearful stress. His body state becomes highly acid, an oxygen deficiency brings on an incurable disease, and he dies.

According to a physician connected with a prison, newly-arrived inmates in general show high blood acidity, but interestingly, in the monthly physical examinations, they find that those who repent and become model prisoners lose that acidity.

When I make a careful observation of such facts, I begin to wonder just what is sickness?

6. Elixir of Life

In the book *Tales From a Western Castle* by Yasushi Inoue, there is a very interesting conversation between Genghis Khan and an invited Chinese scholar, regarding long life.

Genghis Khan: "You come from far off, do you have medicine for long life?"

Scholar: "There is a way of healthful living, there is no medicine."
Genghis Khan: "Then there is really no medicine for long life?"
Scholar: "There is a way of healthful living, there is no medicine."

Germanium regulates the amount of cholesterol in the blood, and by animal experimentation, it has been proven that it prevents amyloidosis, the ring leader in causing the phenomenon of aging. At the 64th Conference of the Japan Pathological Society held in April 1975, the results of the following experiment were presented:

"In ICR mice two years old, spontaneous development of amyloidosis was widely observed in various organs of 12/14 cases, including the kidneys, digestive organs, liver, spleen, heart and adrenal glands. No relationship of amyloidosis with chronic inflammation was established. Mice of the same strain were used as an experimental group. These animals were fed organic germanium from five weeks of age for a period of 22 months. In the 30 mg/kg administration groups, amyloidosis was induced in 3/6 cases. On the other hand, in the 300 mg/kg administration groups, 12/14 cases presented no sign of its development."

Perusal of this report reveals its amazing significance. Amyloidosis, also known as amyloid degeneration, as any medical encyclopedia will tell you, is a disease which occurs when amyloid degeneration appears in the body. In plain words, it is the principal cause of aging. Since organic germanium completely inhibits the development of amyloidosis, it would be no exaggeration to call organic germanium an "elixir of life."

Germanium in the Treatment of Disease in General

The impotence of modern medicine against incurable diseases is simply flagrant. The root of impotence lies in the absence of philosophical background in modern medicine. As a result, it easily falls into an attitude of local or microscopic research; the methods of treatment become symptomatic. For this reason, when cure of cancer or Behcet's disease, for example, by prescription of organic germanium compound is reported, the doctors laugh me off saying, "Are you a magician?" My reply is, "No, on the contrary, the god cast a spell on me to synthesize organic germanium compound from elemental germanium and to use it to treat incurable disease; the magic is in the hand of the god."

1. Methods of Treatment at the Clinic

What distinguishes the germanium clinic from other clinics and hospitals is its methods of treatment. Our Clinic is located in a suburb of Tokyo, where a physician and three other internists work for internal medicine, internal neurology and physiotherapy. In addition, consultations are conducted for geriatrics and general health. Such demarcations of clinical treatment are not essential, but are of some convenience and thus are retained even in our clinic.

I am convinced that only the patient has the power to heal himself through his own efforts, while the doctor merely passes on to the patient his acquired knowledge and the technicalities pertaining to the cure. Therefore, I took pains to stress this point not only to the doctors, but also to the pharmacists and nurses. The doctors in our clinic thus take ample time for consultations, determining the mental attitude of the patients, talking with them about ways and means to overcome their disease, and collaborating with them to find a method of cure. The use of conventional pharmaceuticals hitherto employed in hospitals has been minimized, while the mainstay of treatment has been the administration of germanium.

In my view, based on Oriental medicine, any disease is basically due to the constitutional characteristics of the patient. Of the constitutional characteristics, the blood plays the principal role. The cause of disease probably lies in oxygen deficiency of the body, for the supply of oxygen throughout the body depends on the hemoglobin in the blood; besides, antibodies that grapple with the pathogenic bacteria also exist in the blood. For this reason, we should aim at the blood as a means to cure or prevent disease.

Now, hydrogen of positive ions may be regarded as dust in the blood. This is generated with carbon dioxide after the combustion of food taken into the body system for energy. Carbon dioxide is exhaled. The hydrogen ions combine with oxygen to become water excreted in the form of urine and sweat. An acid blood means an excess of hydrogen ions in the blood, which deprives the blood of large quantities of oxygen, causing oxygen deficiency in the body system. For this reason, acidosis or acid blood is considered the very cause of various diseases. The two important causes of acidosis are food and mental stress. No genuine recovery can be obtained unless these important factors are kept in mind in consultation and treatment. Therefore, the treatments in our clinic have as their integral parts dietary guidance and efforts to remove the stress of the patient.

When our clinic was opened, few patients visited us. However, with the growing achievements through our constant efforts, which have been conveyed to the public by word of mouth, a considerable number of visitors now come to our clinic. I am proud that there has not been a single complaint regarding treatment by germanium alone by those treated who now total several thousands. All those who have cured themselves of their disease are grateful for our method of treatment and continue to take germanium for the maintenance of health.

2. Excerpt from the Director's File of the Clinic

By Dr. Shigeru Makiuchi

Many of the patients visiting the organic germanium clinic have undergone lengthy treatment at university hospitals or national, public or private hospitals, without experiencing any improvement in their condition. In general, they are people who have heard of germanium from friends or relatives who themselves have experienced cures or remissions, or at least an improvement in their respective diseases by the intake of organic germanium.

Gradually, the effects of the organic germanium, sometimes almost bordering on the miraculous, are becoming widely known and recognized, and the number of doctors favoring an "organic germanium treatment" has increased throughout Japan. Accordingly, the number of patients calling on the Organic Germanium Clinic by recommendation of such doctors constantly increases. Unfortunately, however, not a few patients have distorted ideas about this compound. Hence, I wish to clarify some points as a doctor at the organic germanium clinic.

To begin with, organic germanium is now available in different preparations to facilitate its administration in various disorders: (1) in capsules, (2) in granules packed in alu-foil, (3) in injection solution (for hypodermic, intramuscular and intravenous injection), (4) in suppositories, (5) in cream form, (6) in solution contained in vials as a drip for eye, ear and nose.

Regarding the toxicity of organic germanium, the results of tests have shown organic germanium to be nontoxic and completely harmless. These tests on acute and subacute toxicity, deformity and accumulation were carried out by a professor and his research staff at the laboratory of a renowned university and by an authoritative research institute entrusted to undertake this task.

A large number of patients entertain erroneous ideas with regard to the side-effects of organic germanium. While it has been prescribed by many doctors to a large number of patients during the last eight years as a test treatment agent, no side-effects have been observed either clinically or biochemically.

When viewed from the patients' viewpoint, however, symptoms that may be suspected as being side-effects, do appear. Such symptoms are especially liable to appear in patients with liver and kidney disorders, in allergic people, in those who are susceptible to bronchial asthma and hives and in patients suffering from stomach and intestinal disorders, constipation, chronic articular rheumatism and gout.

This is one of the characteristic actions of organic germanium. Toxic elements, products of decomposition, waste matter and foreign matter generated in the body, which are injurious to health or which obstruct disease-curing processes, are discharged with the urine, feces and also through the pores of the skin. In such cases, the volume of urine may increase, the feces may become softer and even watery and the frequency of discharge may increase to several times the usual amount. Unlike the effects generally known as diarrhea, however, no abdominal pains accompany this process. Furthermore, when such matters are discharged through the skin by insensible perspiration, rash accompanied by itching appears. This symptom differs according to constitution, age, diet, duration of disorder, existing condition of disorder and the dosage of organic germanium. Such phenomena are observed more frequently in patients with larger amounts of internal toxic elements. However, since these are the effects of organic germanium, the symptoms disappear within three days to two weeks when administration is in progress or when the dosage is controlled under instruction of the doctor in charge. Having overcome these effects, the patient will feel fine. For example, when a patient suffering from gout or chronic arthritis takes organic germanium, the pain may intensify when the pain-causing substance (uric acid in the case of gout) is removed from the joint, but when administration is continued, the pain will be reduced within a few days to a few weeks. If treatment is suspended because of the pain the administration up to this point will become meaningless.

People with all sorts of ailments visit the Organic Germanium Clinic. Thus, data on countless cases accumulate, a few of which should be cited:

Atopic dermatitis (8-year-old boy, weighing 21 kg): Typical symptoms appeared all over his body a few months after birth. He was examined by specialists at different hospitals, underwent many sorts of treatment, including adrenocortical steroid treatment, without any effect. As later severe itching occurred, he was continually scratching himself. This had given rise to a complication in the form of acute inflammation and rash, swellings, local feverishness and pain became prominent.

Organic germanium was prescribed four times a day—after each meal and before going to bed—at the rate of 20 mg per 1 kg body weight. In addition, germanium cream was rubbed on the affected areas once immediately after rising in the morning and once before retiring at night.

After two months of treatment his condition improved around the elbows and knees, and he stopped scratching himself. Administration of germanium is being continued.

Retrobulbar neuritis (state of total blindness) (32-year-old woman, weighing 50 kg): Her eyesight began to decline about a year ago, and gradually she became almost totally blind so that she could not distinguish between day and night. She underwent treatment at well-known ophthalmic hospitals without any effect.

The patient accompanied by her father was told at the Organic Germanium Clinic that it was doubtful whether any effect could be expected, since all the physicians attending her had given up the idea of cure. On the insistence of father and daughter, who refused to give up, treatment was started orally twice a day, once after breakfast and once after supper, at the rate of 40 mg per 1 kg body weight. In addition, she was told to use one drop of the eye lotion eight times and more per day.

The result was that the patient became able to distinguish between day and night within one month. Her visual acuity improved to 0.1 in two months, to 0.4 in three months and after six months to 1.0. Needless to say, the patient and her family were delighted, saying the improvement was miraculous.

Subacute myelo-optico-neuropathy (SMON) (50-year-old woman, weighing 48 kg): Acute sensory impediment appeared about 15 years ago, and because of a severe motor impediment in both lower legs, she began to experience difficulty in standing upright, walking becoming impossible. Obstruction of visual acuity gradually increased, her left eye becoming virtually blind. She had to use a wheelchair when she came for examination.

The sensory impediment in her lower legs was deep, muscular atrophy and decline of muscular strength became conspicuous and she showed the syndrome of the pyramidal tract. She also experienced urinary incontinence occasionally. On instruction, she twice daily took organic germanium capsules, once after breakfast and once after supper, at the rate of 40 mg per 1 kg body weight. In addition, she was told to use germanium eye drops five times or more daily.

She started to walk again with the aid of crutches in about two months. When she visited the clinic three months later, she was able to walk with only the help of a stick.

Case of Nephrosis Syndrome (80-year-old man, weighing 55 kg): Edema appeared in the lower legs about a year ago, and he was treated at a public hospital for several months with adrenocortical steroid preparation, immunization depressors and others, but the edema grew worse expanding up to the abdomen and chest. It ultimately became an anasarca. Lasic and other diuretics were used, but the edema persisted. When he was brought to the Organic Germanium Clinic he was unable to walk.

Examination showed his total serum protein content to be 5.8 g/dl, serum albumen content 2.7 g/dl, total cholesterol value 310 mg/dl and the urea nitrogen content 24 mg/dl (others omitted).

As the 24-hour value of urine protein could not be measured, the first early morning discharge was measured and showed 300–500 mg/dl. Blood pressure was 190–120.

Organic germanium in capsules was prescribed three times daily to be taken after each meal, in a dosage of 30 mg per 1 kg body weight. However, as the decline in edema was too slow even after two weeks, the dosage was increased to 40 mg per 1 kg body weight, with the same frequency of administration. As a result, the edema began to disappear first from the chest and then from the abdomen, and three weeks later it was only apparent in the lower part of the legs. His weight decreased to 51 kg, and after another two weeks the edema in both legs disappeared completely, while his weight decreased to 49 kg.

Examination of the patient at this stage showed a total serum protein content of 6.1 g/dl, serum albumen content of 4.2 g/dl and urea nitrogen content of 21 mg/dl. The blood pressure was found to be normal. In addition to administration of germanium, the patient remains under observation as to his daily habits and diet.

Case of Cerebellar Degeneration (25-year-old woman, weighing 48 kg): Difficulty in walking and speech impediment gradually developed about three years ago until she was no longer able to walk. Furthermore, she lost the ability to write. She had nystagmus, tinnitus and trembling limbs. Over a period of eight months she went from one specialist to another, to be told at last that she suffered from cerebellar degeneration. However, as the cause for this condition remained unclear she was told that there was no way to help her. When she at last came to our clinic, carried by her father and brother, she was a virtual cripple.

Organic germanium was prescribed orally at a dosage of 40 mg per 1 kg body weight, to be taken twice daily before breakfast and before supper. Within one month her speech impediment gradually declined and after five months her writing impediment, nystagmus and trembling of the limbs decreased. After ten months not only did her speech and writing impediments further decline, but she became capable of rising on her own and was even able to walk a short distance. Tinnitus and trembling had completely disappeared. She continues germanium intake.

Case of Hepatoma (56-year-old man, weighing 66 kg): Symptoms such as loss of appetite, loss of weight, general weariness and abdominal inflation began to appear from early June, 1977. He went for treatment at a hospital, but examination revealed liver cancer which was certified by liver puncture, liver scientigraphy, etc. He came to the Organic Germanium Clinic by recommendation of the hospital doctor in charge of his case. The result of the examination was a clear case of cancer of the liver and spleen, which could be felt at a distance of about six fingers from the costal bow. Abdominal dropsy and anemia were observed, but not jaundice.

Organic germanium, at 35 mg per 1 kg body weight, was prescribed three times daily before each meal. On August 3, the patient carried a letter from his attending physician requesting the doctor at the Organic Germanium Clinic to give the patient a daily intravenous drip injection adding 5% glucose to the germanium solution. In addition to this daily intravenous injection (10 ml injection solution containing 200 mg organic germanium), germanium in capsules in a dosage of 60 mg per 1 kg body weight was prescribed to be taken three times daily before each meal. In addition, one suppository a day was used after evacuation. From September 2, intravenous injection solution was increased to 320 mg per day.

According to a report from the doctor in charge, the patient had been making good progress, when he caught a cold in mid-November accompanied by fever. In early December an estimated 2,500 ml of abdominal dropsy was observed. Under these circumstances the daily injections were increased to 600 mg from December 15, accompanied by an oral intake and the use of suppositories in the same amount as before.

When the patient was again hospitalized on January 13, 1978, abdominal dropsy had disappeared and neither the liver tumor nor the spleen tumor could be tactically perceived. Examination on March 28 showed his condition to be almost normal. The doctor in charge conceded "no medicine that treats cancer so effectively has yet been developed. Moreover, the absence of side-effects is amazing. I am now wondering if it really has been cancer." The followings are the results of the biochemical serum tests (excerpt):

Exam. Item date	July 6 1977	Aug. 3 1977	Oct. 4 1977	Nov. 8 1977	Jan. 13 1978
GOT	157	227	221	162	62
GPT	122	87	81	54	32
Al-P alkaline phosphatase	19.3	16.5	15.8	16.4	14.8
LDH dehydrogenated lactic acid enzyme	490	480	630	552	460
LAP leucine amino-peptidase	240	155.8	156	152	156
γ-GTP gamma globulin protein	50.3	42.0	21.0	17.0	17.0
S-Cu serum copper	222.7	172	157	138	129
α FP alpha-fetoprotein	75.2	94.0	63.0	30.4	23.0

3. Cases Taken from Clinic Records

The following examples are selected from the case histories recorded at the Clinic to illustrate the efficacy of the organic germanium on diseases generally considered incurable.

Case 1 (Behcet's 42 years old, male, farmer): The patient had been suffering for about five months from failing eyesight and difficulty in walking when he was admitted to a public hospital, where he was diagnosed as having Behcet's disease. The treatment at the hospital did not bring relief, and his condition steadily deteriorated. He had to be helped by two persons when he was brought to our clinic in a desperate condition.

We had had several previous cases of that disease which could be healed by the administration of massive doses of germanium. The doctor sent him home with a 20-day supply, instructing him to take 1.5 g daily. He was also given careful instructions emphasizing the importance of a correct diet and mental attitude.

Ten days later he telephoned the clinic, reporting that his eyesight had begun to return and that his general condition has been improving daily. On the 20th day he came for an additional supply of the germanium compound. He was a completely different person.

There are three other cases of Behcet's disease where the compound showed a marked, or at least some efficacy.

Case 2 (Hepatic dysfunction, male, 30 years old): The organic germanium has a remarkable efficacy on liver troubles as shown in the subjoined figure. The patient had been suffering for more than three years from serum hepatitis caused by blood transfusion. He was constantly returning to hospitals. The ineffective treatment caused severe depression.

Treatment with the organic germanium has completely cured his ailment as attested by a doctor recently, although it took 2 years.

As shown in the thin horizontal line in the figure, the normal values of GOT and GPT are within 30 units (10 to 40 units for GOT). In S's case, these values rose in May, 1972 despite the treatment with germanium, probably due to the fatigue caused by the transfer of his place of work.

The percentage of recovery among patients with cirrhosis when treated by administering germanium is considerable. This is particularly noteworthy in view of the fact that this disease is regarded as one of the most difficult hepatic troubles to cure. Let us note here that more than 10 patients with cirrhosis have already escaped death through our germanium therapy.

4. Two Examples Using Organic Germanium

(i) Apoplexy. One day an elderly man about my age who lived just behind me, was suddenly stricken with apoplexy and was unconscious. Immediately a physician practicing in the neighborhood was called but since there was no way for him to administer oxygen, he could only stand there with his arms folded. The man's son came running to me for help, and I gave him a solution of my germanium

A case History of Hepatic Dysfunction (S, 26 years old)

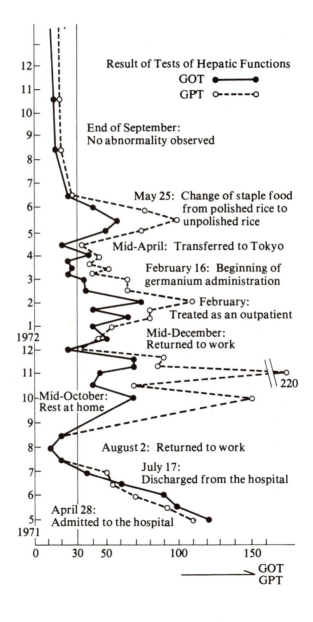

and showed him how to give it by mouth or through a tube inserted in the nostril. After a few hours the man regained consciousness and was able to talk. The next day he could get up and go to the bathroom by himself. To every one's amusement, that very day the same physician saw him and cried out, "It's a ghost."

In those days I told everyone that in case a person suffered a stroke of apoplexy or had softening of the brain, he should be given my germanium within six hours by mouth if possible or through a tube in the nose.

By this means two firemen were saved from carbon monoxide poisoning just short of death. A construction worker at the point of asphyxiation was also restored to life.

Whenever things like this happen, the doctors are amazed and wonder if I am not using some kind of magic. Because of all these things, I urge old men with a fear of apoplexy always to carry germanium on them when they go out.

(ii) Raynaud's Disease. One day I had a visit from a lady who once was a popular movie star and is now active as an instructress of traditional Japanese dance.

The lady began telling me of the severe pains in her fingers and toes she had been experiencing for quite some time. She had been consulting a number of physicians who invariably told her that a cure could hardly be achieved. Hearing that her illness was diagnosed as Raynaud's Disease, I could understand the physicians' reactions, for with this disease limbs get befallen by gangrene and in its advanced stage it requires the amputation of the affected limb. Fortunately I could tell her that there had already been 4 patients in our Clinic with this particular disease who could be cured with germanium in a relatively short time. I followed up this information by offering her a water solution of germanium in a whisky glass while explaining that germanium increases the oxygen supply to the body which would help to cure the disease. Suddenly I found myself being eyed very angrily by that lady who insisted that what I had just given her to drink was nothing but an alcoholic drink. In spite of my refutation and assurance that it was germanium, she insisted that it must have been alcohol, for she had begun to feel warm all over just as would be the case when she would have had some liquor. I replied "That is only an evidence that germanium has already started showing its effect. I am only surprised at the surprisingly quick response." Only a few minutes after this incident she suddenly exclaimed "Look at my hands, Dr. Asai! They have turned pink!"

While sitting opposite her it was the color of her hands that first caught my eye which were of wax-like paleness. Now the overall feeling of warmth and well-being seemed to have spilled over into her hands, for they showed a very intensive pink and one had difficulty thinking of them as belonging to the same person who just a short time ago had these sickly pale hands.

Another surprise was in store for us, for when she rose to leave she had no difficulty in walking and she insisted that the pains in her feet were gone and she actually refused the help of her two attendants who had accompanied her to my house.

Ten days later she related how she had enjoyed a walk with her husband. That stroll was the first after a long period of invalidity. Her happiness showed also in her voice which sounded extremely youthful.

5. Efficacy on Eye Diseases

I sometimes am reminded of the blind patients that often came to my office. There were diseases of the retinal blood vessels, such as glaucoma, black cataracts, detached retinas, inflammation of the retina and optic nerves, and without exaggeration, I can say that it was amazing how effective germanium had been. I often witnessed scenes where patients wept as they cried out, "Now I can see!" Those who could not see would invariably say, "If I could only see again, Doctor, I would give anything. If it were money I would even go into debt to pay for it. I cannot understand the psychology of people who know the joy of seeing, and yet do evil things and are greedy. There can be no greater happiness in the world than being able to see..."

During the International Angiological Congress, I met a professor of ophthalmology at the State Medical College of Rio de Janeiro.

He wrote that using the germanium compound on a patient virtually blind with amaurosis yielded amazingly good results, and that the patient was well on the road to recovery. It had already been verified that germanium rejuvenates retinal vessels, and is therefore effective in treating glaucoma and amaurosis. His letter has added new evidence of its efficacy.

6. Efficacy on Hypertension

Extensive experiments on animals and clinical tests have demonstrated repeatedly that organic germanium has excellent efficacy on hypertension and cardiac disorders.

Organic germanium compound was administered to a rat with induced hypertension and its blood pressure dropped to normal level. Moreover, when administration was continued, this did not cause a further drop in the blood pressure as would be the case with depressants. On dissection a marked difference was observed between the heart of the rat to which the compound was administered and that of the control rat. The heart of the rat to which germanium was administered revealed no morbid distension, while its surface was red, glossy and live in appearance. The heart of the control rat was generally blisterous and a dirty gray color.

Hypertension is one of the most common and troublesome diseases that beset us today. Organic germanium may be regarded as an excellent agent for treating this disease because of its efficacy on the disease and lack of such side-effects as those found using existing depressants.

In July 1972, I participated in the International Angiological Congress held in Rio de Janeiro and read a short paper reporting the remarkable efficacy of the organic germanium compound on hypertension. During the meeting I was appalled to learn that no remedy without any side-effect had been found for hypertension. One German doctor explained to me, "Hypertensive patients are likely to die at any moment, it is as if they were carrying a live bomb in their body. Therefore, they use depressants despite their harmful side-effects because they think liver or heart troubles caused by the side-effects are still preferable to succumbing completely."

This really shocks me. Nevertheless, such a logic is accepted in modern medicine because modern medicine primarily attempts to make symptomatic treatments.

"I have heard," I told my audience, "that if one takes a depressant too often, this will do more harm than good because depressants lower the blood pressure excessively, aside from their other ill-effects. In striking contrast, an overdose of the germanium compound will produce no such harmful effect. It will lower the blood pressure to the normal level, but never below that level. On the other hand, when it is used on a case of hypotonia, it will raise the blood pressure to the normal level." The reaction of my audience was that of disbelief, but it only strengthened my conviction that at present the germanium compound is the only remedy for hypertension.

7. Effect of Germanium on Glands

Germanium has a beneficial effect on glands in general; a pathologist friend reported that all mice to which the germanium compound was administered had an increased weight of their secretory glands, (endocrine organs), especially the adrenal and thyroid glands. They became a reddish color, indicating blood viscosity had decreased, thus facilitating blood flow.

As for rejuvenation of secretory glands in humans, there are a number of cases on record of 50 and 60-year-old women long into their menopause, resuming menstruation. Several others spoke of relief from pains and anxieties normally accompanying climacteric disorders. Numerous cases of marked improvement or recovery from uterine cancer are on record at the clinic, including uterine myoma, breast cancer, and bladder cancer among others. Cancers in the reproductive organs have been medically determined to be due to disorders of the adrenal hormones, and the most widely practised method of treating cancer of the prostate gland is the administration of female sex hormones, while adrenal glands are removed in treating breast cancer.

One day I went to the clinic and found the whole staff holding their sides in fits of laughter. This began after a woman past 50 had come in and told them the following story.

"My abdomen ached so I went to the K hospital for an examination, and was told that I had a myoma as big as a fist in my uterus and would have to have surgery. I had to wait ten days for a bed, and thinking to increase my body strength, I began taking copious amounts of germanium. After ten days I went back to the hospital where surgery was scheduled for the next day. The following day I was prepared for surgery and taken to the operation room. There the doctor made a final examination but the tumor he had declared to be as big as a fist could not be found. The doctor was sure that they had brought in the wrong patient, but his check-up proved that I was the one all right. So I just got down off the surgical table, leaving the doctor with a very puzzled face."

Administration of the germanium compound in advance will restore these organs to a state of health, preventing the occurrence of such disorders.

An old man of 75 years was suffering from an enlarged prostate gland. The doctors at a university hospital repeatedly urged him to have surgery, but he continued to refuse since his health in general had been fundamentally sound. His condition worsened until finally surgery could not be delayed.

The old man recalled that two years before he had visited me, and remembered my germanium. He wrote from Kyoto and asked if germanium might be effective with his prostate problem. I wrote that if he would take 800 milligrams of germanium every day he would not have to have surgery, and sent him a supply by special delivery. With a cheerful voice he told me that it was no longer necessary for him to have a tube inserted in order to pass urine. Being able to urinate freely as of old was to him the best thing ever. "Thank you," "thank you," he cried, and I could imagine him bowing repeatedly before the phone, as he expressed his great joy. A week later the doctor said he was completely healed and needed no operation.

Germanium seems to rejuvenate the adrenal glands of the internal secretion organs.

8. Experience with Organic Germanium: Dr. Takahiro Tanaka

Dr. Takahiro Tanaka (Chofu Hospital) who has been using the organic germanium compound for treating his patients reports:

"Before attempting to use a new substance for therapeutic purposes, I always try it myself first to determine its efficacy and side-effects. For testing the organic germanium compound, I took from a 500 ml water solution containing one gram of organic germanium a daily dose of 20 ml (equivalent to 80 mg of organic germanium), divided in two portions, one in the morning and the other in the evening, avoiding simultaneous intake of any other drug.

I was then nearly 60 years old, and had complaints of general languor, enervation, a heavy feeling in the head, and a pain in the prostate gland.

The intake of the germanium compound had the following results:

(1) Within one or two days after beginning the intake of organic germanium, languor and the heaviness in the head disappeared and I began to feel full of vigor.

(2) I began to have an erection on waking in the morning and my sexual appetite returned.

(3) The pain in the prostate gland was alleviated and eventually disappeared.

(4) I began to have regular stools in heavy quantity every morning and lost nearly 10 kg of weight over two months to a standard weight level.

(5) I slept soundly and required less sleep.

(6) Complexion improved and the chilly sensation in the limbs disappeared.

(7) Small, red itching eruptions appeared dispersed on the skin of the head and the back.

A marked rejuvenating effect was observed. The itching eruptions described in (7) were the only side-effect, which subsequently was noticed in 2 to 3 per cent of study cases, but was invariably transient.

On the strength of these findings, I used organic germanium for treating cases of cancer, including post-operative patients, arteriosclerosis, cerebral apoplexy (brain hemorrhage, thrombosis, softening of the brain), sequela of cerebral apoplexy, climacteric disorders, heart troubles (angina pectoris), stomach ulcer, depression, epilepsy, senile mental diseases, chronic rheumatism and Raynaud's disease. Except for stomach ulcer, organic germanium showed a marked or some degree of efficacy in almost all cases.

NOTABLE CASES TREATED WITH GERMANIUM

For post-operative treatment of cancer (female, 61 years old): A thumb-sized malignant tumor was discovered in the right cervical region 15 years ago, and was removed subsequently. Three years after this excision, the patient underwent an operation for removing a gland cancer on her left breast, followed a month later by a similar operation on the right breast. Another malignant tumor was found again on the right cervical section, which was removed. Soft tissues and lymphatic glands around the cervical tumor could not be removed. Radiation treatment and anticancer agents were not used. A daily dose of 800 mg of organic germanium was administered. Over three years since then there has been no sign of recurrence.

The cervical tumor was histologically diagnosed as a gland cancer which appeared to be a lymphatic metastasis, but no primary lesion was observed. Although the case history had an excision of cancerous tissues in the same cervical area 13 years ago, which leads me to suspect a latent slow-developing malignant tumor, no recurrence has actually developed subsequently.

Arteriosclerosis, cerebral apoplexy and sequela to apoplexy: I am convinced of the efficacy of the organic germanium compound in these diseases in shortening the time required for recovery. In some cases, however, concurrent administration of cytochrome and other agents proven to be effective made it impossible to attribute the efficacy solely to organic germanium.

Heart diseases including myocardial infarction: The time needed for recovery was shortened through treatment with organic germanium.

Case C (66 years old) suffered from sclerotic heart disease for which there is no effective medication, symptoms being pain in the chest, bradycardia, and slow pulse. On administration of the organic germanium compound the patient soon felt relief from the chest pains, and although he had difficulty in walking, he recovered enough to be able to ascend a slope without frequent rests.

Organic germanium proved effective also on angina pectoris. Its administration to a case where coronal dilators showed little efficacy brought relief within a couple of days, reducing the frequency of attacks which were two or three times a day to almost nil. In another case of angina pectoris, attacks recurred upon ceasing the administration of the organic germanium compound.

A case of Raynaud's disease (male, 45 years old): The patient had his fourth toe amputated at a hospital. A black gangrene developed at the amputated part, while the third and fifth toe were pale due to poor blood circulation. The black gangrene increased despite the administration of 1400 mg of methyl carbamate and peripheral blood vessel dilators. Therefore, 80 mg of organic germanium compound was given. Three days later, the gangrene was markedly reduced in size and the pale toes had turned rosy with good blood circulation, showing signs of gradual recovery.

After a month, the patient began drinking and smoking again. The dosage was not increased. Probably this negligence caused aggravation of the gangrene and the lower leg was amputated. It is to be noted, however, that before the gangrene became worse, the administration of organic germanium showed a remarkable efficacy in improving the symptoms.

A case of hypertension, stomach ulcer and arteriosclerosis (male, 72 years old): The patient was admitted to the hospital with many diseases. A thumb-size niche was found in the angular part of the stomach, from which copious bleeding occurred. A severe case of anemia ensued, which at one time was measured to be 31 per cent in hemoglobin concentration by Shal's method, while the red blood cell count showed 1,700,000.

Transfusion of blood and other fluids, and administration of various hemostatics performed daily failed to bring about any relief. If more than 50 ml of blood was transfused, the excess blood would be discharged with urine. Therefore, blood transfusion was limited to 30 ml, which left the patient in the worst possible condition.

In addition to blood transfusion, 40 mg of royal jelly was injected every other day. This treatment resulted gradually in a slight improvement. The patient unfortunately suffered a great mental shock by a conflict in his family, causing a senile mental disorder in the patient who in the height of confusion went so far as to throw his feces around. Then, 80 mg of organic germanium compound was given to him.

When examined by X-ray fluoroscopy, the large niche had disappeared and the stomach ulcer had nearly healed, leaving a scar. On the 10th day of administration of the organic germanium compound, the patient suddenly recovered from his state of confusion.

9. Experience with Organic Germanium: Dr. Okazawa

By Dr. Mieko Okazawa, Ooka Clinic of the Infant Protection Association, Social Welfare Corporation

When we see people with bodies no different from ours fall ill time and again, we cannot help uttering words like "you are so frail". We utter "so frail" with a deep sigh, yet we are not sure on what basis we distinguish between "frailty" and "robustness." Such is the discordant mental state with which we challenge diseases. As a pediatrician, one often feels like criticizing obstetricians and gynecologists, the doctors who handle the cases prior to the pediatrician, for not doing this or that.

The body that develops, for instance, cholecystitis is more easily susceptible to cystitis, pyelitis and chalazion of the eyelid. Such a person is subject to constitutional diseases of one type or another without any conscious action. A person with such a "body" is at a disadvantage throughout his life.

A person with a constitution subjected to repeated illnesses, a person handicapped by such a poor body or a person with a so-called "allergic constitution" ultimately falls victim to some obstinate disease of unknown cause. When one comes face to face with such a person, one feels the urge to help him, but the greater the urge the more one feels the importance of keeping the body of the mother in the best possible condition prior to the birth of that person.

This is a very natural hope requiring no urging by a woman doctor like myself, and it was organic germanium and its properties that have fulfilled this hope. In the world of nature where amphoteric ions are at work, the action of germanium borders on the miraculous.

Anyone who hears of organic germanium for the first time associates it with its inorganic form, a nonmetal, thus causing needless concern. It is not enough that it does not accumulate in the body; if coming into contact with the dreaded "cation" of heavy metal accumulated in the body, its "anions" are said to combine easily with the former and discharge will take place in the form of urine and feces. In this respect, the research work of Dr. Asai leaves no doubt as to its authenticity.

As to the strong action of organic germanium, some specialists suggest the presence of some invigorating element other than oxygen, but the fact that it does invigorate, may mean that anion-oxygen indispensable to internal organs in itself is more than sufficient for human vitality.

When I personally came across organic germanium, I felt that this was what I had been looking for in my work as a physician whose aim it is to help people overcome the afflictions with which they are cursed. I still remember vividly the emotional impact this realization had on me; successive experiences were proof that my initial impression had been right.

People who have resorted to the intake of large doses of organic germanium or who made long-range use of small amounts in order to improve the condition of their internal organs, find their formerly pasty-colored skin turn to a healthy complexion. Expressions of agony on their faces disappear. In children, their faces brighten and their eyes regain their sparkle; the faces of adults become serene, their hope for recovery returning. As to aged persons, the odor peculiar to the aged, stemming from poor metabolism, disappears.

People will tell me with wonder among other experiences the disappearance of warts, the outgrowing of corns and splinters embedded in the skin, healing of eczemas and healing of burns without scars with little of the accompanying pains resulting from those burns, or of early subsiding of herpes. While this shows the effectiveness of organic germanium in minor ailments, later descriptions will deal with its effectiveness in much more severe and obstinate diseases. If people experience only small effects, if any, this only goes to show that their condition is worse than thought, thus an increase of the prescribed dosage is required. Where the body' cells lack oxygen, so indispensable to life, a gradual decline in bodily functions is inevitable and lastly the fire of life will be extinguished.

This is my personal opinion, but it seems that forces working towards the improvement of health and forces working towards an aggravation of physical conditions are in constant struggle within our bodies, and the condition improves or worsens depending on which of the forces gains the upper hand. What is commonly applicable to all cases is that prescription of large doses of organic germanium immediately after a definite diagnosis brings wonderful results.

Nothing, no miracle drug nor mysterious recipe, prescribed in haste after the condition deteriorates will bring the expected results, if the envigorating capacity of oxygen within the body is lost.

Being cured of a severe disease should not lead the patient to overestimate his regained strength: the convalescence period might range up to a year or more. Contraction of a disease difficult to cure means that forces that work towards an aggravation of that condition are much stronger than those working towards recovery. To prevent worsening of the condition, or rather to prevent a return of the disease, care should be taken to continue the prescription although at a reduced dosage, while efforts should not be overlooked to maintain the normal potential within the body.

A phenomenon that occasionally bothers patients who are prescribed organic germanium could best be explained as a cure reaction (deceptive phenomenon in Chinese medical herb therapy) which causes a certain condition to become worse. This, however, should not cause additional anxiety but rather be judged as a sign that the treatment is beginning to have an effect. In such cases it is necessary to increase the dosage for a certain period (between 7 to 14 days) in order to overcome this phenomenon. The larger the dosage, the quicker will be the breakthrough.

For instance, in the case of articular rheumatism, the hips and the knee joints become so painful about the 7th day after beginning the administration of large doses that the patient will be unable to leave his bed. The phenomenon will be the more severe, the worse the condition of the patient. However, when the dosage is increased when the phenomenon occurs, the patient will be free of acute pain within about three days, and it will not be long until he can walk again.

After passing through this period, the continued intake of a reduced dosage will lead to gradual improvement, with an occasional return of the cure reaction in a lighter from, a process which I like to call "shedding of the disease."

In the case of stomach ulcer, hematemesis or melena may take place at some stage after beginning administration, but as this is a cure reaction, a breakthrough can be made by increasing the dosage; this also applies to cases of piles. This phenomenon of cure reaction, therefore, should be taken as a sign of efficacy.

This is the beginning of a chance for cure, and it is most inadvisable to suspend administration by mistaking the condition for a sign of aggravation. This is the most important junction, and good mutual understanding between the doctor trying to cure and the patient wanting to be cured is essential.

In conclusion, I shall cite various examples of clinical treatment I have given.

Case of Cerebral Thrombosis (female, 78 years old): She had been suffering from headaches and a sensation that her shoulders and neck were in a vice, a condition in cerebral thrombosis. A month after prescription of organic germanium both the oppressive feeling around the neck, and the headache disappeared completely. The dosage was reduced subsequently, and she now, after nine months, leads a normal life.

Cases of Hardness of Hearing (females, 85 years old and 70 years old): The first case had had trouble in hearing for twenty years, but six months after prescription of germanium, she was able to hear the ticking of a wrist watch. Now she can lead a normal life without the use of a hearing aid. The other woman has improved now to the extent that she can hear children's shouts which was not possible before treatment.

Case of Cardiac Infarction (male, 45 years old): One morning he had an attack of sharp pain in the chest. As his electrocardiogram was known to be abnormal, a large dose of organic germanium reserved in advance for emergency use was administered. The agony subsided in a few minutes and he fell asleep (about three minutes after the onset of pain). The electrocardiogram taken after he had had a nap showed extremely high St. Administration of large doses continued and the ECG showed an astonishing improvement by the third day, as shown by the following figures:

GOT (149 at the time of attack) → GOT (11) after 3 days
GPT (60 at the time of attack) → (18) after 3 days
MG (8 at the time of attack) → (4) after 3 days
ALP (7.7 at the time of attack) → (5.9) after 3 days

Now, he is able to work quite normally. However, he constantly carries organic germanium in his pocket for emergency use.

Cases of Mental Disorder: As it is not always possible to expect a patient's voluntarily expressed wish for treatment, it is for those around him to urge him to take the drug under a long-range program.

An example is the case of a patient with mental disorder, a condition generally accompanied by an unfavorable constitutional make up, in this instance obstacles affecting internal secretions. By stabilizing this condition the patient cheered up and was capable of returning to normal social life. With self-confidence restored he appeared to be an entirely different person.

In the case of a 15-year-old girl, she was diagnosed as being in the early stage of schizophrenia. She became autistic, began to distrust everything and to absent herself from school. One month after prescription of organic germanium, her menstrual pains disappeared, her facial expression brightened and her personality became very cheerful. She returned to school after one year's absence.

As mental cases are usually allergic to various things, they are highly sensitive to the effect of germanium. The sensitivity, however, is not in an undesirable direction; they feel the effect even of small dosages pleasantly. For this reason, it is as well to prescribe small doses first and then to increase them gradually in accordance with their initial reaction to germanium.

Case of Autonomic Ataxia (female, 35 years old): Such afflictions occur surprisingly often in people of this age. Symptoms include apprehension, cold extremities, physical instability (giddiness), heavy feeling in the head, insomnia, palpitation of the heart and depression of unknown causes. Patients in a serious condition are hospitalized, while those in a worse condition are referred to a mental hospital. When organic germanium was prescribed for a patient who claimed that the medicine prescribed at the psychiatry department made him feel worse, the feeling of heaviness in the head disappeared, physical instability was gone and mental orientation returned in ten days. She also began to sleep better, and when administration was continued at a reduced dosage for the following year, she recovered enough to forget the various symptoms that had caused her suffering.

Case of Whiplash Syndrome (male, 48 years old): He complained of headache, stiff shoulders and pain in the arm as a result of a traffic accident that took place ten years previously. However, 18 days after organic germanium was administered three times a day, he was free of pain. He continued to take it for six months thereafter.

Case of Articular Rheumatism: Many people complain of pain in the joints. Such cases are found in particularly large numbers among women past middle age. Cases concerning elbow joints, shoulder joints and finger joints are comparatively easy to treat, but cases involving knee joints have a much more difficult time because of the walking movements.

A feeling of pressure and acute pain develop around the knee joints and hips for some time prior to manifestation of the signs of improvement after prescribing organic germanium. The patient at this stage is temporarily confused thinking that his condition has worsened. However, if the dose is increased at that time, the pain disappears, RAT that has been plus turns to minus in about three days, and the patient will be freed from pains suffered for many years. In the case of articular rheumatism, an especially large dosage is desirable in order to shorten the period of suffering. The prescription can be continued in reduced dosage after relieving the acute pain.

If a large dosage is not possible in the treatment of articular rheumatism, exercise, such as walking up and down stairs many times a day, speeds up germanium's effect, leading to earlier liberation from the pain that sets in at the turning point towards improvement, and to a lightening of the load felt on the lower limbs.

Case of Pneumonia (female, 86 years old): Large doses of organic germanium were administered because of severe coughing and high remittant fever. This was continued for seven days, but in consideration of her age and need for reinforcement of vitality, the dosage was reduced to half and continued. Full recovery has been achieved. Cases of pneumonia increase in winter, but in the four years since the use of organic germanium began, no cyanosis has been experienced and no hospitalization for pneumonia has been necessary. This state is entirely due to the efficacy of germanium.

Case of Asthma: Asthma attacks all age groups. Intake of organic germanium when the fit occurs inevitably relieves breathing difficulty, and the larger the dosage the quicker the relief. Although there are differences depending on the seriousness of asthma and individual physical make-up, about six months is enough to see the patient's complexion improve, a disappearance of the suffering from his face and of the dropsical swelling.

A Case of Asthma (female, 41 years old): The patient was constitutionally weak with such complaints as asthma, hypertension, headaches, constipation, pains from abdominal adhesion, hypersensitivity to pharmaceuticals, general itches as well as liver and kidney disorders. She had been taking Chinese herb medicines for two years but little improvement had been obtained. On April 15, 1974, the patient was persuaded to undergo administration of organic germanium at least for six months regularly. Initially a dose of 20 ml was given twice a day, and the dosage was gradually increased to 40 ml taken once a day, although divided into three to four times a day when the patient suffered pain. Within a month of administration the patient took a total of 6,000 mg (500 ml × 3 bottles) and began to feel better, relieved from headaches and enjoying good general physical condition. In May of previous years, she used to complain of physical disorders, but this year she felt so well that she declared she was no longer ailing. Although she suffered from headaches before rainy days, pain from abdominal adhesion and itches had all disappeared.

In the sixth month, relief was obtained from pains of asthma, headaches, insomnia, lumbago and constipation that had persisted for many years. After a year of continued administration, the remaining complaint of hypertension was also stabilized to a level between 140 and 90. The patient now enjoys good appetite and is in good spirits.

Cases of liver cirrhosis, esophageal varices, abdominal dropsy (*Ascites*) —(In many of these cases diabetes mellitus complication is found. As these are very obstinate diseases, administration of large doses from the beginning is desirable.)

Esophageal varices gradually collapse and become scars (when esophageal varices break, bloody feces are discharged). This may be noted from around the tenth day of administration, but need not be of concern as this is the turning point towards improvement. Abdominal dropsy also subsides and assumes the (−) state. In this case, a large dosage hastens recovery. If the patient responds speedily, the abdominal dropsy (ascites) disappears in one month, and a stabilized condition is reached in about six months. Even when all is well after a year, prescription of organic germanium should be continued as long as possible because of the nature of disease. If the patient should catch cold, contract some new disease or develop fever, a larger dosage should be given, otherwise, complications may develop or the disease under treatment may become aggravated.

A case of diabetes, liver cirrhosis and esophageal varices (male, 63 years old): The patient had been suffering from diabetes for 25 years. In March, 1973, he vomited blood caused by liver cirrhosis and esophageal varices. Admitted to hospital, he awaited surgical intervention on the esophageal varices.

On May 21, the patient began taking 40 ml of water solution of the organic germanium compound three times a day.

On the 8th day of administration, the abdominal dropsy began to disappear.

On the 19th day, the liver function also began to be restored, and the patient was discharged from the hospital at his own request. (The dosage was increased to 80 ml three times daily.)

On the 30th day, some blood was found in excreta due to contraction of the varices. The dosage was reduced to the original amount, but the patient was in good physical condition with a good complexion and able to walk about.

In the fourth month of administration, most of the varices examined by esophagoscopy at the hospital presented a whitish surface, and no longer was rupture feared, with only one varix near the stomach remaining greenish. The dosage was increased again to 80 ml, which after three days resulted anew in blood in excreta.

After sixth months, upon examination at the hospital, the varices were diagnosed as healed, and the patient was allowed to take any food and to lead a normal life.

Cases of gastric ulcer, gastritis: These cases also occur in large numbers. In these cases, too, the stomach begins to feel heavier at the turning point towards improvement under administration of organic germanium. When the dosage is increased at this time, the feeling of oppression disappears in three to seven days. Subsequently, administration is continued in reduced dosages, and the treatment may be stopped when the patient recovers to the point where he does not even notice that he has a stomach. If he takes germanium as soon as he feels something wrong with his stomach at any later date, his stomach will become normal at once.

In the case of gastric ulcer, it is important to increase the dosage at the turning point instead of suspending administration thinking that the condition has become aggravated. If the disorder is serious, it will take longer to reach the turning point.

In addition to these cases that have been successfully treated with organic germanium, there are numerous notable cases in which the efficacy of organic germanium has been demonstrated. These include: a case of general stiffness (causes unknown) that was cured in six months; two cases of hyperthyroidism that showed an improvement in the course of treatment; cases of pneumonia in infants or influenza with such complications as pneumonia, bronchitis, diarrhea, etc., recovery from which was early.

10. Guarding against the Effects of Pollution

It is an understatement that much has been said and written on the subject of world pollution. Particularly relevant here is pollution of the air and of foodstuffs. This contamination gradually builds up in the body and can lead to very serious diseases. For instance, there has been a long-continued use of mercury and cadmium in fertilizers etc., that in sufficient amounts can lead to metal poisoning.

To study the efficacy of organic germanium on mercury poisoning, I asked a pathologist to use it on animals. At the time, the shocking symptoms of mercury poisoning cases of people who had eaten mercury-contaminated fish in a particular area of Japan were widely reported, and there was a real sense of urgency to relieve the plight of the victims.

The experimental results obtained by the pathologist were as I had expected:

"An intravenous injection of 0.6 mg of mercury chloride to a rat weighing 200 gm induced a calcareous deposit in the cortex of the kidney 20 hours after the injection. A high degree of calcareous deposit was also observed in the medulla.

The rat was then treated with the organic germanium compound, and after 10 days, most of the calcareous deposits disappeared, and after another 20 days, no trace of calcium was observed. The dead cells were found dispersed, some of them in the interstices of the tissues. After 30 days of germanium therapy, these were replaced by healthy cells, thus showing the efficacy of the treatment.

Moreover, another experiment in which mercury was given to a rat along with germanium compound revealed no toxic symptoms in the rat. Thus, germanium administration appears to have an adequate effect in preventing mercury poisoning."

Once I had samples of my hair analyzed to determine the mercury content. The average mercury content was 0.98 ppm which showed that methyl mercury harmful to the living body was virtually nil. The available data on the mercury content in the hair of inhabitants in Tokyo on the other hand gives the following figures:

Average inhabitants: 6.9 ppm (17.7 ppm max., 2.6 ppm min.)
Those having a heavy intake of fish: 12.0 ppm (19.3 ppm max., 4.7 ppm min.)

It is generally agreed among investigators that the mercury content in the hair of Japanese ranges from 5 ppm to 10 ppm. Since harmful organic mercury accounts for 70% to 80% of the total mercury content, these high figures for the mercury content in the hair among the Japanese are alarming. If the methyl mercury content in the hair exceeds 20 ppm, danger signals show in such symptoms as abnormal perception, difficulty in walking, and loss of normal visual ability, and if it exceeds the 30 ppm mark, the mercury poisoning may be fatal. The mechanism of poisoning by methyl mercury has not yet been fully clarified, although one hypothesis is that the properties of mercury atoms and the free organic radicals that combine with them

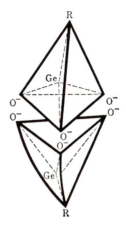

cause an electrodynamic disturbance in the living body.

Upon request similar experiments on animals were conducted using cadmium instead of mercury to determine the effects of germanium on cadmium poisoning. The data obtained clearly indicated the efficacy of the germanium compound.

The best method of solving mercury or cadmium poisoning is simply the prevention of accumulation of mercury or cadmium in the body through constant discharge or a therapy which captures and discharges any amount if accumulated.

The structure of my germanium ideally suits it for this task. The organic germanium compound has a cubic structure with three negative oxygen ions around germanium as shown in the subjoined diagram.

The negative oxygen ions are at the base of the cubic triangle. Two cubic triangles whose bases face each other make a molecule.

Any heavy metal accumulated in a living body is in a state of positive ions which would jump into and be trapped in the mesh structure of the negatively-charged oxygen ions of the organic germanium compound taken into the body.

The germanium compound with its semiconducting properties is discharged completely from the body about 20 hours after its intake. On its way it not only captures any heavy metal accumulated in the body but discharges itself with it from the body. So long as we live in this polluted environment called Earth, we are bound to succumb in the end to pathological changes in our body and mind caused by contaminated food and air. If pollution and invasion of contaminated substances into the body are unavoidable, the only escape seems to me the cleansing of these substances from our body, or making our body resistant to contamination. I am convinced that the organic germanium compound will play a role in achieving this solution.

I touched upon the efficacy of organic germanium in removing contaminated food from the body when describing its efficacy in metal poisoning. In this respect polybiphenyl chloride PCB has to be mentioned, the toxicity of polybiphenyl chloride appearing when its chlorine combines with the biphenyl radical to become organic chlorine. If this chlorine is separated from the biphenyl radical to make it inorganic chlorine, it will lose its toxicity and be discharged from the body. Various means of detaching the chlorine from the biphenyl radical are conceivable in modern molecular chemistry; for instance, radiation may be utilized. The organic germanium compound appears to have a special electrochemical action. In a chemical experiment, a phenomenon which can be regarded as evidence of its action to separate the chlorine has been confirmed.

The fact that organic germanium compound orally administered is absorbed by way of the intestines into the blood where it combines with blood cells to circulate through the body has been pathologically confirmed. Consequently, its remarkable efficacy has shown itself in the liver, lungs and brain cells where the blood influx is heavy.

11. Efficacy in Children

One of the striking features of the organic germanium compound is its invariable efficacy on children. For example, a three-year-old boy suffering from a brain disease called "ligated circle of Willis" considered by modern medicine to be extremely difficult to treat was cured completely, after only a comparatively short period of administration of germanium, so that he could go to a kindergarten.

My two-year-old granddaughter contracted acute otitis media and kept crying with pain. We could relieve the pain by giving her 40 ml of water solution of germanium compound and the effect was obtained in about 10 minutes. Twice more she was given the same dose and the following morning, a copious discharge of pus from the ear occurred, the swelling subsided and she recovered quickly.

In addition, the quick efficacy of organic germanium has been demonstrated in such cases as toothache, empyema, alveolar pyorrhea, infantile asthma, and infantile nephritis.

Progressive muscular atrophy and mongolism are among the most horrible of diseases that affect children. Organic germanium has shown at least an inhibitory effect on their progress. Further study is required on the massive dosage required.

No less horrible are extensive burns in children. In such cases, cure can be obtained in an unbelievably short period by applying an ointment containing organic germanium to the affected area along with oral administration of the germanium solution; to be noted is that the burn heals with hardly any scar. The efficacy is similarly great on chilblains.

We have found another remarkable effect of organic germanium on children. My grandchildren taking it regularly proved to be nearly immune to influenza. In addition, when German measles played havoc in their kindergarten, my grandchildren were not affected. The teacher in charge telephoned their mother, warning her to take special care of her children, because the teacher thought their immunity was due to an abnormality in their constitution.

The following two examples are taken from the Clinic records: *Patient after operation for congenitally blocked bile duct* (6-month-old boy, weighing 7 kg): After birth his condition was thought to be the usual jaundice, but as the condition became aggravated, he was examined by a pediatrician who then advised an operation because of the probability of a congenital disorder. It appeared the child had an advanced case of cirrhosis.

As soon as he was discharged from hospital, the parents on advice of the doctor brought the child to the Organic Germanium Clinic.

Examination showed severe jaundice, overswelling of the abdominal wall veins, liver tumor, spleen tumor and abdominal dropsy.

At first, organic germanium in granular form was prescribed four times a day—morning, noon, evening, and at bedtime—at the rate of 60 mg per 1 kg body weight. The granules were either dissolved in water or milk for administration.

As no change was observed after two weeks of administration, the dosage was increased to 100 mg per 1 kg body weight and given six to seven times a day. During the three weeks since then abdominal swelling, overswelling of abdominal wall veins and jaundice have improved, though slightly, and the patient has regained vitality. The treatment is being continued.

Guillain-Barre-Syndrome (3-year-old boy): In June, 1977, the boy abruptly complained of stomach ache and pain in the lower legs. At the hospital to which he was taken his case was diagnosed as probable acute cerebellar ataxia. Repeated examinations, however, showed it to be a case of Guillain-Barre-syndrome, and since it was in a progressive state, there was no special treatment. He could stand when holding onto the bed, but walking was difficult since his knees gave way so that he easily lost his balance. He also began to experience urinary incontinence. When he was brought to the Organic Germanium Clinic in early July, he was unable to walk and complained of pain in his abdomen and lower legs.

When granular organic germanium was administered three times a day at the rate of 600 mg per day, the boy became capable of walking within a week. In addition, in a report received from the parents in early September, it was stated that the boy was walking normally and was playing in the neighborhood, although his tendon reflexes were still a little weak. In November, four months after the first visit to the clinic, he was found to be no different from any normal boy, although he was easily prone to loss of balance. Still, it was thought safe to reduce the intake to a daily 300 mg which he will continue to take for some time.

As a result of published work, I have had mail from many people. Their words and enthusiasm have encouraged me. It is not an exaggeration to say that these letters pile up like a mountain, and each line in them, whether telling of suffering or overflowing with joy, touches my heart.

I will select one about a child, written by his mother; she writes, "There are no doubt others having the same trouble, so for their sake. . . ." With her permission I am passing it on, not in the original with its many pages, but only the most important portions.

My son is in the sixth grade of primary school. Last year he had pneumonia which left his body weakened, and now when catching cold, it would continue for a long time. When his temperature would not drop I gave him antibiotics to reduce the fever. He often stayed away from school, and when he did go, there was so much homework assigned that his health broke as a result and he had to continue resting.

In the early part of March he had a fit which came upon him about an hour after he had gone to bed. He talked deliriously, his body shook, and his mind seemed to be confused. There was some difference in severity, and in duration, but generally, after that, about an hour after going to bed, he was sure to cry out and his body shake. I was alarmed and took him to the doctor I had gone to when he had the cold.

I explained the situation, and he took an EKG, and sure enough there was an abnormality. He told me to keep a diary, and every two weeks come for medicine which he prescribed. The fits continued unchanged, so he prescribed a stronger medicine and in larger doses.

My son took the medicine morning and evening, but seemed to become drowsy, and yawned during the day. He became languid, and always took a nap as soon as he came home from school.

The doctor himself was not sure what was wrong but wondered if it could be epilepsy, night terror, or loss of coordination in the autonomic nerves.

The child's progress was failing before our very eyes.

Then, one day at a Chinese herbalist's, I happened on a pamphlet from the Organic Germanium Clinic. I did not understand all the theories, but almost like a flash there came the feeling, "This is it!"

I went to the Organic Germanium Clinic, and under the doctor's instructions began administering germanium. I had him take the germanium in the morning and that day there was no seizure. Day after day I sighed with relief, 'Ah, another day and nothing happened.'

As you advised me, I did not worry unduly, and was very careful of the diet. I stopped using the medicine from the hospital. Over a week passed with no seizures, and the boy declared, 'I feel like doing something, I feel good,' and his expression was one of vigor.

His recovery was so fast that I grew careless, and forgot to give him his germanium. In the morning he took his sun bath, did his school assignments, and read his books, but apparently he overworked his eyes and brain, and in the afternoon went to bed. We were all worried, but when I gave him his germanium, his pain seemed to leave him immediately.

By such neglect, was it possible that the blood vessels in the brain became constricted, and an oxygen deficiency or anemic condition resulted?

There is one other thing I want to tell, you. From the time his fits began, he either was tired or lacked strength due to the cold and always had to rest during the school's physical exercise period. After starting to take germanium, of his own accord he began taking part with energy and will.

When the school had gone on excursions, I kept the boy out lest he be a bother to the teachers or the other students, but with this change I felt it would be alright, and sent him along without any worry.

What words can I find to express my appreciation.... A most hearty thank you!"

All the foregoing examples show that organic germanium has a far more remarkable and quicker effect on children than on adults. In my view, its efficacy on adults is inferior to that on children be-

cause of the following three factors:
1) Deterioration of the constitution due to the strain and stress of modern living and environment,
2) Deterioration of the constitution by intake of contaminated food,
3) Morbidity of the constitution of Japanese exposed to excessive and indiscriminate use of pharmaceuticals.

My view is supported by the fact that organic germanium has shown a remarkable efficacy on adults who could avoid the above three factors. These factors lead to acidification of the body fluids, and thus to oxygen deficiency.

Clinical examples of the amazing effects of germanium on children have been succesively reported to me. I am overcome with joy at the prospect that children could be freed from the agony of disease. The following two clinical examples have been reported by Dr. Mieko Okazawa of the clinic attached to the Infant Protection Association mentioned earlier.

A case of difficulty in walking due to nervous overstrain (girl, five years old): The patient was forced to study very hard to pass the entrance examination for a prestigious private primary school. The overstrain incapacitated her from walking and she was admitted to Hospital K. A dose of 60 ml containing 240 mg of the organic germanium compound in water solution was orally administered, divided into 20 ml portions to be given three times a day. In the second week, the patient recovered enough to be able to walk again. She was completely cured one month after the beginning of germanium administration, and full of regained vigor, she successfully passed the entrance examination of the private school. She continues to take the germanium compound daily, morning and evening.

A case of influenza complicated by pneumonia (male, 1.5 month old): The baby contracted influenza infected by members of the family all of whom had come down with this epidemic. It ran a fever of 38.2°C and its cough showed the symptoms of pneumonia. Initially the germanium compound solution was administered two or three times a day, 10 ml each time; with increasingly frequent coughs 10 ml of the solution was orally given 10 times a day and 20 ml was injected five times a day. In addition, fomentation with mustard was repeatedly applied.

On the seventh day of administration, rales were marked in the chest and the cough continued. On the eighth day, however, the course suddenly turned for the better with hardly any rales or coughs, and on the 10th day, the baby was well again.

Weighing only 2,730 g at birth, the infant did not seem to have sufficient resistance, but thanks to the massive administration of the germanium compound the cure could be accomplished.

Dr. Okazawa spoke of the efficacy of germanium in children as follows:

"We treat many infants and children. Every year when influenza is rampant, some infants are bound to contract pneumonia. Then we face an acute shortage of oxygen tents. Nonetheless, with the advent of organic germanium, its administration to infants has enabled us to cure them without needing to send a single infant to an oxygen tent."

Similar reports on the remarkable efficacy of germanium have been received by me from various sources. I can therefore claim with conviction that the organic germanium compound is indispensable for treating infants and children.

12. Germanium and the Mind

If you consult a medical encyclopaedia regarding mental disease, you will find a large number of terms describing particular types of disease, which may be largely classified into the congenital types and the acquired types. Their causes are usually not clearly indicated. What is certain is that these diseases are related to the brain.

Among the various organs of the human body the highest level of oxygen consumption occurs in the brain. The brain consumes 20% to 30% of the total oxygen supply to the body. According to the medical encyclopaedia oxygen consumption by the brain is often governed by its supply to the brain and is closely related to the blood flow to the brain.

Assuming that the thinking faculty hinges on the oxygen consumption of the brain, a better oxygen supply would improve this faculty. It is known through measurement of brain waves that the consumption of oxygen by the brain increases during higher mental activities such as thinking and working on mathematical problems.

The organic germanium compound in the bloodstream plays the same role as oxygen, and therefore increases the total amount of oxygen in the body. This is attested by the following report made by the biochemical laboratory of Tohoku University, Japan:

"An experiment was conducted on the effect of the organic germanium compound on oxygen consumption in the liver and diaphragm of a mouse. The result indicates that the germanium compound inhibited the consumption of oxygen."

The amount of oxygen supplied is closely related to the blood flow, which in turn is related to its viscosity which decreases with the increase in the amount of oxygen available. As the viscosity declines, the blood flow eases.

Administration of the organic germanium compound decreases the viscosity of blood considerably. Consequently, organs such as the liver and adrenal glands where the blood influx is high, increase in weight, a fact confirmed in animal experiments. From this it can be deduced that taking the compound will increase the blood flow to the brain, thereby increasing the oxygen supply to that organ.

I am inclined to believe that various types of mental disorders are caused by an oxygen deficiency due to a disorder in the blood circulation in the brain. This view is based on the fact that relief can be obtained to an almost dramatic extent just by supplying sufficient oxygen through administration of the organic germanium compound. Thus, I have succeeded in relieving many from the complaints accompanying softening of the brain, manic-depressive psychosis, hysteria and even the after-effects of whiplash injury. Among those helped are promising young men who are now pursuing their respective paths full of vigor, which fills me with indescribable joy and happiness.

Softening of the brain (female, 70 years old): She was confined to bed. On the seventh day of administration of a daily dose of 3,000 mg of the organic germanium compound in water solution, she recovered enough to take meals. Two months later, she could walk about the house.

The efficacy of the organic germanium is pronounced in this particular disease. Its effect is remarkably rapid when administered at the onset of symptoms. This disease is caused by defective blood vessels which prevent oxygen supply to the brain. The efficacy of the organic germanium which accelerates the oxygen supply is therefore naturally to be expected. The same applies to cerebral thrombosis.

It is to be noted in passing that mere inhalation of oxygen or injection of ozone cannot bring about the effect mentioned above. Such inactive oxygen must have its ions activated by enzymes in the body to have any effect.

The organic germanium compound, on the other hand, plays the same role as oxygen in the body, so that its oxygen supply can be retained without being completely consumed, which indeed is the essence of life.

13. Treatment of Depressive Psychosis

By Takahiro Tanaka, M.D., Head Physician, Chofu Hospital, Chofu City

I. INTRODUCTION

In 1973, I had the chance to report on organic germanium, the carboxyethyl sesquioxide of germanium developed by Dr. Kazuhiko Asai, used in the treatment of diseases in general.

Since then, I have observed many cases which has enabled me to verify the efficacy of organic germanium in a variety of diseases, of which I refer in this report in particular to cases of depressive psychosis. On occasions, I am afraid, some statements may not convey the full meaning since I am an internist and thus less knowledgeable about psychopathy.

The number of patients suffering from depressive psychosis, including those with manic-depressive psychosis, whom I had the chance to attend during the eight years since 1970 and who are covered in this report, amounts to only seven or eight. Furthermore, only five of these were treated with organic germanium for periods long enough to justify reporting. Under these circumstances, it may be presumptuous of me to make this report, but, being an internist who has only very few antidepressants at his disposal, and thus having no alternative but to use organic germanium for treatment, has allowed me to evaluate objectively the efficacy of the compound in specific diseases.

II. CASES

Case 1 (reported previously, female, 27 years old): In 1971, when still a university coed, she suffered from depressive psychosis following appendectomy. It was four days after the occurrence of the symptoms that I saw her. The patient's eyes appeared vacant and were full of tears, typical symptoms of depressive psychosis. Administration of 80 mg organic germanium per day was advised. Within two days, the patient's eyes became alert, the appearance of vacancy and misery being dispelled. Another two days later, her complexion had returned to normal and hardly any speech impediment remained. Ten days later the patient accompanied by her mother went for a three-hours train ride to attend the annual examination at her university.

In this case, the total dosage of organic germanium taken during the days of treatment was 2 g, *i.e.*, 80 mg per day, after which administration was discontinued. Two to three times during the said period Diazepam was also given. A dose of 5 mg of this was given before bedtime because she complained of difficulty in going to sleep.

Seven years have now passed without a recurrence of the observed symptoms.

Case 2 (male, 38 years old): On January 16, 1975 the patient experienced a second seizure of depressive psychosis. It was one week later that a member of his family came to consult me; at that time he was an outpatient at a psychiatrist's office. At the next visit I noticed his vacant eyes and his lack of speech; he was under the influence of Tofranil. According to the psychiatrist it would take about two months for him to recover from this bout. I prescribed organic germanium, 100 mg twice a day, to be taken in the morning and in the evening. A week later, although he still complained of intense languor, his eyes appeared much brighter. He was instructed to reduce the Tofranil dosage to half the present amount. Two weeks later, his eyes had returned almost to normal, and after another month he returned to work. He continued the intake of organic germanium for nearly one year. Although three years since the onset of the second seizure have elapsed, no sign of a recurrence has been observed.

Case 3 (reported previously, female, 58 years old): Since 1968, she has had repeated periods of depressive psychosis at intervals of six months. While in the beginning these lasted for up to three months, each recurrence worsened her condition, until it reached the point of attempted suicide in 1970. At that time she began organic germanium treatment. She had been suffering from persistent insomnia and had been taking 10 mg doses of Diazepam when unable to sleep. Being pampered and stubborn, she very often spurned her family's advice of taking the drug, thus being awake all night.

Since no data were available as to the use of organic germanium in the treatment of depressive psychosis, I was not sure whether giving it in this particular case would produce any results. Within two to three days after beginning the intake of 10 mg twice a day, mornings and evenings, the persistent insomnia had lifted, while the symptoms of depressive psychosis had almost vanished. The intake was continued for another three years. It is now almost eight years since the last bout. No problems have been observed since then.

Case 4 (female, 69 years old): She has a history of 30 years' depressive psychosis. The bouts would occur in a set pattern, the symptoms appearing with the advent of the cold season, lasting through May and gradually disappearing towards the summer. She would continue to feel well till the onset of the next cold season.

Starting in November, 1973, she began taking organic germanium in a water solution (2 g dissolved in 500 ml water) that would last one month. The daily dose would consist of 70 mg in a divided dose, taken before meals in the morning and in the evening. The administration continued until the summer of 1976, during which period no further attack occurred. In July 1976, probably because of a sense of ·relief of being freed from all the trouble, the patient discontinued the intake of the compound and continued to feel well all through the rest of that year. Then, in January, 1977, she had to undergo an operation on a cataract in her right eye, the consequence of which was a relapse into the former symptoms. In August, 1977, the patient resumed the intake of organic germanium, 100 mg per day. Soon, signs of improvement became visible and the patient was again able to sleep through the night. She is in good health today.

Case 5 (female, 70 years old): More than 30 years ago the patient began to suffer from depressive psychosis, said to have started when she had to evacuate to the country.

In this case, a bout of the depressive state would last for three months, followed by one month of well-being before her condition would turn to a manic state for two months. This pattern would be followed by quite normal behavior. When I saw her, however, symptoms had become quite unsteady, a depressive state today would be followed by a manic state tomorrow. Usually, the depressive state was dominant in January and February. It was on January 14, 1977 that she began a daily dose of 100 mg organic germanium. During January all went perfectly well. In February, mild symptoms were noted but subsided within about 10 days. All through March, April and May her well-being continued, a state not felt for years. Confirmedly, she became less careful with the prescribed intake, particularly since April, often skipping the intake for a day or two and, when going on a trip in May she forgot to take the powders with her. After her return the symptoms reappeared. Being stubborn, she refused to accept the advice of her family and her doctor. At last the administration was suspended.

14. Attendance at the World Congress of Natural Medicine

The World Congress of Natural Medicine is an organization of scientists who will not conform to modern medical practice, and their first meeting was held in Aix-en-Provence, an ancient capital north of Marseilles, France. Specialists in harmony with the principles of the organization gathered from all over the Western World. Similar meetings have been held since in Biel, Switzerland and in 1977 in Florence, Italy.

Since I had repeatedly insisted that my organic germanium did not belong to modern medicine but was nearer Chinese herbs, I too was invited to the meeting. The first meeting of the congress, made up of some 200 kindred spirits, opened in Aix-en-Provence. The lectures were translated simultaneously into English, German, and French so their content could easily be understood by all. There was excellent rapport between the lecturers and the audience throughout the three-hour sessions.

As already noted, the congress was made up of scientists who had misgivings about modern (Western) medicine and therefore many of the presentations dealt energetically with Eastern or Oriental therapies such as acupuncture, massage, iridology, ion therapy, homeopathy, and vitamin therapy. In addition, a number of lectures dealt with the treatment of cancer by means other than those used in modern medicine. As one contributor said, "Fed-up with poisons and the ineffectiveness of modern medicine, scientists are promoting herbs, or acupuncture, or diet, or electrotherapy, but there are limits to their properties. Especially, there is a feeling of helplessness in the case of the incurable diseases. But organic germanium has broken down the wall wonderfully. Men have toiled long years to develop natural therapies, but this marvelous product seems to crown them all."

Another said, "When used along with Chinese herbs a double effectiveness will show up, and with acupuncture, or electric therapy, germanium will provide marvelous healing powers. It is the same with iridology, looking at the iris may help discover the malady, but after that dieting may be the only treatment. With the coming of germanium, we have something of great concern to iridology."

15. In Conclusion

Letters of gratitude from people who have been suffering from Behcet's syndrome, SMON disease, aplastic anemia, sarcoidosis and incurable hepatitis, which Japan's Ministry of Welfare designates as incurable diseases, fill the files in my study. Here is one short note of gratitude from an 86-year-old woman living in Yokohama, Japan, who had chronic asthma, white cataracts, was hard of hearing and passed her days in darkness.

"Since I have learned about germanium, I have had no more pneumonia, I can hear, and now I am able to read my favorite books again." She enclosed this verse:
> My umbrella grows heavy day by day
> But germanium helps me carry on.

Each letter is an indictment against modern medicine and a record of people who have found new light in life amidst intense suffering.

Just as a small candlelight can be seen from afar in the dark, the fame of my work on the organic germanium compound appears to have reached far corners of the world. Thus numerous letters imploring to obtain the compound are pouring in from such countries as Switzerland, Germany, Australia, Romania, Canada, and the U.S.A.

Whatever the outward signs and symptoms there is a cause for every sickness—a deficiency of oxygen in the human body.

After a dose of organic germanium, within a short time the amount of oxygen in the body is not only greatly increased, but dehydrogenation takes place, and poisonous matter is rendered nonpoisonous, and in about 20 hours is thrown out of the body. Since germanium does not remain in the body, there is absolutely no toxicity, and no harmful side-effects that occur with all medicines. When I say that germanium is effective against all sickness, I can imagine not only doctors but people in general laughing and saying I must be joking.

In fact, it *is* proving effective against all diseases, and I believe the doctors are going to have to reverse their ideas of medical practice, and treat sickness on a holistic basis, since it deals with the whole nature of man and his life environment.

I am convinced that this organic germanium compound promises to be more important than any other drug, and its study requires a long period; in spite of the cost research should be continued for the benefit of humanity.

Germanium in the Treatment of Cancer

A Chinese proverb says, "Better to light a candle than lament the darkness." Darkness still prevails in the world regarding cancer and other obstinate diseases. I am attempting to keep a candle alight with the organic germanium compound.

1. A Challenge to Cancer Cells

I have dwelled on aspects of the treatment of diseases of the body and mind in general in the previous section and now I intend to concentrate on that disorder that may affect all parts of the human form, cancer. Once again, bearing in mind for a moment the fact that oxygen is the source of life for all living things, it is all the more understandable how harmful an oxygen deficiency can be. The internationally famous German scientist, Dr. Otto Warburg, clearly states in his thesis on cancer that the growth of cancer cells is due primarily to cellular oxygen deficiency. Since the normal, healthy cells in our bodies are aerobic, an insufficient supply of oxygen alters the structure of these cells which develop a series of abnomal reactions in order to survive under such conditions. The cells begin glycolysis and turn anaerobic. The nuclei of cells which have undergone such changes are exact replicas of the nuclei of malignant cancer cells.

An article taken from the Nov. 8, 1973 issue of the *Medical Tribune*, seems to support the Warburg theory on the ulceration of cancer. It continues to the effect that the theory has met with objections from various quarters, but a number of prominent researchers do support it saying that cancer can be controlled by preventing oxygen starvation from occurring in the cells. Waltenburg, of the University of Minnesota, also agrees with the theory by saying that antioxidation drugs can inhibit the formation of lung cancer. Indeed, using our organic germanium compound in 20 patients with lung cancer there has been almost 100% recovery.

Related also to the above theory is a recent discovery made by Professor Hans Selye of the Faculty of Medicine at the University of Montreal. Prof. Selye revealed that if the amount of blood flowing into a living organ is reduced slightly by lightly binding one of its blood vessels, the organ will develop a state of morbidity. Reduction of the blood flow reduces the supply of hemoglobin by which oxygen is supplied, thereby producing an oxygen deficiency with morbidity as a consequence.

Another clue to understanding the nature of cancer as a particular disease is to think of disease as a certain state of the human being who is nothing more than an organic mass. Understanding of the nature of man, therefore, is essential to treating any disease. Having tackled the question "what is matter?" within the range of limited human knowledge, modern physics has confirmed that man is an aggregate of minute electrically-charged particles. In terms of modern quantum physics, therefore, a disease is interpreted as a "distortion" developing in the aggregate of electrically-charged particles that are close to electrons. That is why electron dynamic action is needed for correcting the "distortion." Herein is found the area where germanium, a typical semiconductor element, plays a vital part.

The electrons of the germanium atom have unique properties that are not found in other atoms. Of its 32 electrons, any one of the four in the outer shell will tend to leap out of its orbit when approached by atoms of other substances—it is by taking advantage of this feature that the electronics industry has been able to use germanium for amplification in transistors, and for rectification in diodes.

The living body is a mass of minute electrical particles and each organ of the body functions as its own concentration of mass of these particles. Accordingly each has a predetermined electrical potential of its own. Since disease results if this potential is disturbed (the potential of a diseased organ being different from that of a healthy organ) the potential of the afflicted organ must be restored to its normal level to effectively cure the disease. It is by employing an effect in the body similar to its semiconducting effect used in electronics, that the germanium compound serves to return this potential to normal and hence cure a disease.

In cancer, for example, it is known that the potential of a cancer cell is markedly different from that of a healthy cell. The potential at a cancer cell wall is high and varies greatly—a factor which may be attributed to the fact that cancer cells multiply at such a rapid speed. The germanium compound, whether administered orally or injected, deprives cancer cells of electrons, and thereby reduces their electrical potential. In biochemical terms, this means that the germanium compound brings about a dehydrogenation reaction, ultimately suspending the activities of cancer cells. It is also by this mechanism that it acts to prevent metastasis.

Other data have established that when the germanium compound is taken in sufficient amounts, radiation sickness as a result of irradiation treatment can be prevented. Radioactive rays, which are gamma rays, emit electrons which destroy cancer cells and tissues. Unfortunately, at the same time, these rays destroy red and white blood cells as well, and have been known to cause the death of patients undergoing prolonged exposure. Recent data have indicated, however, that the atoms of the germanium compound securely fasten to red blood cells and shelter the cells from oncoming electrons by diverting them around the atom.

Another effect the germanium compound has exhibited in relation to cancer and other diseases, and which may be attributed to its semiconducting characteristic, is that it completely kills pain: pains after operations, toothaches, headaches, etc. Pain acts as a sort of a warning given to the brain. Electrons are relayed via nerve cells from the origin of the pain and are conveyed to the brain where they are sensed as pain. Conventional anesthesia serves temporally to inhibit the movement of electrons so that we do not feel pain, and the germanium compound, given in sufficient quantities, also does so, as its semiconducting action stops the movement of electrons

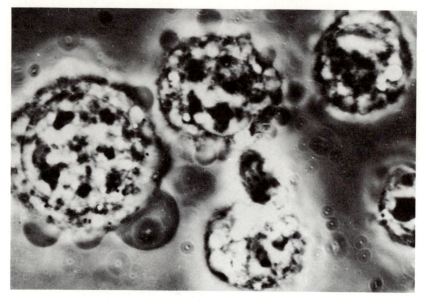

A considerable change in Ehrlich ascites tumor cells under the influence of the germanium compound.
(seen under a phase contrast microscope)

through nerve cells. Unlike anesthesia, however, continuous, prolonged administration is possible due to the absence of side-effects.

Speaking of the absence of adverse side-effects for a moment, it may be said that this feature adds one more note of praise which can be heaped on the use of semiconductors in medical treatment. Physiologically, it is very convenient that germanium is a semiconductor and not a metal, a feature which eliminates the danger of its accumulating in the body. The blood and various cells, having semiconducting properties of their own, repel germanium because of their inherent electrical properties. In fact, one of the major problems now facing our laboratory is that the present compound is discharged so quickly from the body that extensive efforts are being made to produce a compound which will remain in the body for a longer period.

At this point it is difficult to explain scientifically all the medical properties of germanium. Today, there are tens of thousands of medicines in use and not one of them utilizes semiconductor properties. I believe they will come to play a major part, and in fact, bring about a revolution in medical treatment in the future.

2. Prevention of Metastasis

It has long been held by cancer researchers that cancer can be cured if the primary lesion is eliminated. This is not as simple as it sounds, however, as cancer cells mix in the bloodstream and metastasize or migrate throughout the body. Doctors working with the germanium compound have repeatedly confirmed, however, that patients receiving the compound have shown virtually no metastasis. This alone is tremendous news in cancer treatment since, if metastasis can be prevented, cancer can be stopped with a massive attack on the primary lesion.

Although it is known that the dehydrogenating action of the compound has an inhibitory effect on the growth of cancer cells and plays an important role in halting metastasis, precise details of its mechanism are not yet known. One important clue, however, is provided by Dr. Haruo Sato of Tohoku University (Japan), an authority on the metastasis of cancer. In a paper which he presented to the Japan Society for Cancer Therapy, he relates that cancer cells that have entered the bloodstream continue to move with the blood flow. If a pathological condition should develop in a blood vessel, they will adhere to the wall of the vessel, eventually infiltrating and destroying it to proliferate outside. Secondary tumors can be prevented if action is taken to prevent the cells from adhering to the vessel.

Based on Dr. Haruo Sato's theory, a plausible explanation of how the organic germanium compound functions to prevent metastasis is that the increase in the body's supply of oxygen brought about by the compound sharply reduces blood viscosity, thereby improving the blood flow. From a hydrodynamic point of view, cancer cells as an alien substance will continue to flow with the blood without being pushed aside until they reach the capillaries, where they are oxidized and destroyed by the dehydrogenating action of the compound. This explanation is hypothetical and is still being tested, but is not improbable in the light of the activity of the germanium compound.

Information gleaned from our laboratory experiments and clinical observations lend heavy support to the theory that cancer develops due to cellular oxygen deficiencies. Indication is that the high efficacy of the compound in treating lung cancer and liver cancer may be attributed to the activity of the germanium compound in the entire bloodstream flowing through these areas.

In one experiment, a group of five mice were given a hypodermic injection of cancer cells after administering a water solution of the organic germanium compound. Another group of five mice were given a hypodermic injection of cancer cells without administering the solution as a control. The hypodermic injection of cancer cells is a method of inducing cancer in mice generally practiced in the Cancer Research Institute.

The mice injected invariably developed cancer, except those five mice to which the germanium compound was also administered who failed to develop cancer.

This experiment was repeated twice, with the same result.

3. Experiences with Lung and Prostate Gland Cancers

A 54-year-old company employee was diagnosed as having cancer of the lungs. X-rays showed a large bean-size cancerous growth in two places on the right lung. Although he had been injected with anti-cancer drugs, he had lost his appetite and his strength was deteriorating steadily. It was at this stage that he visited the germanium clinic. After ascertaining the details of his case, doctors prescribed a 500 mg daily dosage of the germanium compound. An X-ray photograph taken five weeks later showed absolutely no trace of cancer. In addition, the dry cough peculiar to lung cancer was gone, his overall condition improved rapidly and he soon recovered his former state of good health. There are at least 20 cases of lung cancer at this point which have followed a similar course to complete recovery.

It is difficult at this stage to make an objective assessment of the overall effect or the potential future effect of germanium in the

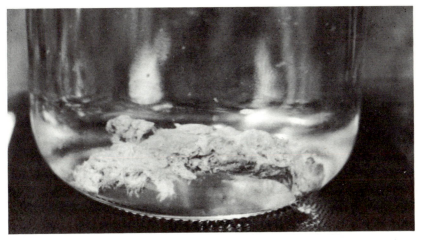

Necrotic cancer cells in the bladder estimated to be discharged through urination after desquamation by administration of Germanium. (From the clinical examples)

treatment of cancer. Its efficacy is not confined to lung cancer. Numerous cases of recovery from various other cancers are on record at the clinic today and results achieved thus far are enormously encouraging. Aside from the fact that the germanium compound stops the activity of cancer cells and halts the growth of tumors, its most promising characteristic is the capability of halting metastasis, or the spread of cancer cells.

For other types of cancers results have also been encouraging. A 62-year-old man complaining of difficulties in urinating was diagnosed as having an enlarged prostate gland, cancer was suspected, and an immediate operation was proposed. The man, shocked at the suggestion of having to undergo an operation came to our clinic and asked if something could be done to spare him an operation. Our doctors prescribed a 0.5% concentration of germanium compound solution in a daily dosage of 100 ml, or a total 200 mg daily dosage. Ten days later, the man reported that his urinating difficulties disappeared on the second day of treatment and he had a healthy appetite.

4. In Praise of Germanium in Lung Cancer

This report of the efficacy of germanium in lung cancer is part of a letter to me:

"The germanium you sent me was used on a 12-year-old girl who had two spreading cancers in her lungs. At the present time the girl's condition is good, and the symptoms of the cancer are gradually disappearing.

The little girl's father fought like a tiger for the life of his daughter. For instance, he took her for an examination to the most famous specialist in Romania. The girl's mother is also a physician, and could appreciate the effectiveness of the germanium.

You will be interested, I am sure, in the results of the treatment since November of last year.

    a. Germanium was given for 3 to 4 days.
    b. Then it was discontinued for 9 days.
    c. Then one gram was given daily for 14–15 days.

After that the same cycle was continued. Up to March 1st, the little girl took 70 grams of germanium. This was bought by Mr. Popa, who, I think, has already sent you a report of this little girl whose name is Alina.

The girl's father would like to learn from you whether he should give a large amount of germanium till she is healed, or should continue till a certain amount has been given, or whether he should continue giving it at all.

If you can give us any kind of a detailed report, I am sure it will mean the sustaining of the little girl's health. We will be most happy for all the advice you can give us."

In a drawer of the desk in my study, in a beautiful envelope is a last will and testament.

Nine years ago (1971), a couple came to my home. He was a young man 35 or 36 years of age. His head was thickly bandaged, his face was blistered as if by fire, and swollen, his skin was very rough, and his color quite dark. He was a pathetic spectacle, unable to look straight ahead, and his wife had to help him to a chair. The following ensued:

"Dr. Asai, my name is Sato. Last year in the spring, I developed a severe hacking cough, and occasionally spat bloody sputum, so I went to the Tokyo University hospital for an examination. The diagnosis was lung cancer in an advanced stage, and I had an operation that removed my left lung. The cancer spread to my right lung, and since I could not have further surgery, I was given injections of a recently-developed anticancer medicine. Very soon all the hair of my head had fallen out, the skin on my face and limbs had swollen up, I felt all the time like vomiting, lost my appetite completely, and felt it would be much better to die than to suffer so much. I thought the doctor could not help me and went home. While I was in the hospital, a man in the next bed asked me to try Dr. Asai's germanium.

'I have come for help.' "

I then told the young man to listen carefully to my instructions, which were as follows.

First of all, he must have absolute faith in germanium, with firm conviction that with it he was going to cure his own disease. Then it was most important that stop all other medicines. Next, he must regulate his diet strictly. When one starts taking germanium, a good appetite is regained and overeating often occurs. For a time he must avoid meat, especially pork, and animal fats. Animal organs such as liver are taboo.

He must change from polished to unpolished rice, avoid white sugar, except, perhaps, just enough for cooking. He must think of a lot of sugar in his coffee or tea as a poison. Fish foods in general are not bad, but he must stop eating eels, and oily tuna.

Here are the things he can eat in quantity: The representative protein foods such as *tofu* (bean curd), *natto* (fermented soy beans), and other bean varieties, vinegar, *umeboshi* (dried and pickled plums), raw vegetables, and sardines. He need not become overly strict, and may eat lean beef occasionally. The main thing is to avoid that which makes the blood acid. If the blood is acid, germanium's action becomes sluggish.

Finally, he must keep in mind that it is he himself who effects the cure, and no one else. His most effective instrument in curing his disease is germanium. With it, the greatly enriched supply of oxygen in his body would do wonderful work. There is no greater tool than this.

Ten days later the wife came for more germanium, and on inquiry I learned that the husband who had been unable to sleep, now slept soundly, his appetite had returned, and he felt fine. He had gone to the hospital for an X-ray examination, and found that the shadow of the malignant tumor had grown smaller. They were most happy.

From the wife who came regularly every 25th day for germanium, we had this report. He was making good progress, and the next X-ray examination after three months showed absolutely no trace of cancer. The doctor who did a biopsy said that while it must be recognized that the cancer had healed, they could not say the healing was complete until after five years.

Just a year later in the spring of the year, I received a fat letter from Sato. In it was a will and two pictures along with a letter. The pictures were of a man rowing a boat at the seashore, with a child of about five riding with him. The figure in the boat had a full head of hair, and face full of vigor. He seemed like an entirely different person.

In the letter that accompanied the will were these words:

"I feel that I am a very lucky man. If it had not been for germanium, I would not be in this world today. Certainly, just as you said, germanium is different from other medicines. After taking germanium I felt life beginning to stir in my body. Living joy like a spring seemed to gush forth in me.

Every time I went for my regular check-up, it was amusing to see the doctor who did the fluoroscope examination shake his head in bewilderment. Truly I am a man who had crossed the line of death. I am as one who has been in Hades and returned.

More than anything else, I have an appreciation for what it means to be alive. My thinking may be immature, but I cannot help feeling that man's life in addition to being controlled by material things, is under the direction of a higher destiny.

What is the value of a man's life? Said simply, is not man's true life value found in saving other men, and living a life of gratitude?

When I received that sentence of death from my doctor, I wrote out my will. Since I will not need a will for some time to come, I am sending it to you for a keepsake."

The reason that organic germanium is so effective in lung cancer is that when it enters the body, it unites with the red corpuscles in the blood, and is thus carried to the whole body, and with all the blood passing through the lungs, the effectiveness there is particularly high. The same is true with the liver, kidneys, and the brain where the flow of blood is especially great.

This accounts for the complete healing of Mr. Sato's lung cancer, previously described, which after eight years with no recurrence, even the doctors have to acknowledge.

5. A Patient's Struggle with Cartilage Malignancy

It is hard to describe the personal struggle as well as the joy on recovery of the many who have been treated with the germanium compound just by recording sheets of clinical data. For this reason, I have included the following story of a cancer patient suffering from cartilage malignancies (chondrosarcoma) which he has recounted from his personal records.

NOVEMBER 1960

I received diagnosis from a major private hospital in Tokyo of having developed a cartilage tumor in the left heel. Shortly after, I was admitted for amputation of my lower left leg.

OCTOBER 1970

Although several years had elapsed since the initial occurrence of the disease, I received further diagnosis at this time of having developed a cartilage tumor in the right lung. The doctor said it was a metastasis of the one removed 10 years ago. A lobectomy of the middle and lower lobes of the lung was performed.

MAY 1971

I decided to begin treatment with natural medicines to ward off any further occurrence of the disease. Shortly after beginning treatment with natural medicines, however, a further report from the hospital showed that a thumb-size tumor had already developed in the remaining portion of the same lung.

To reduce the swelling, I began treatment by taking a mixture compounded of various herbal medicines (*Houttuynia cordata, plantago asiatica, glechoma heder acea subsp. gradis, artemisia, capillaris, licorice and lithospermi Radix*). Supplementing this treatment I also took, separately, molidine, vitacargen, essence of corbicula, and ginseng. Two months later, however, this treatment still had not brought any results. From July to September, I tried cold and hot stimulation therapy, but also to no avail. Home treatment with a Demiger therapy apparatus also brought no results.

NOVEMBER 1971

On the advice of a doctor at the Clinic, I began fasting treatment at a center in the mountains of Central Japan. In conjunction with fasting, I underwent photo-therapy and finger-pressure therapy. I also tried treatment with an electric vibrator during the second week of fasting. After four days the tumor seemed to have grown rather than to have diminished in size.

JANUARY 6, 1972

Met with the Chairman of the Human Medical Association. He advised: "Disease is not the cause of a man's death. It is his persistence in living a life in disaccord with the laws of nature. Illness develops as a warning that one's life-style has gone astray, offering him a chance to change course."

I began to live on a gruel made of pearl barley, fresh vegetables, soybeans and seaweed. In addition, I took a mixture of five major herbal medicines (enzyme, sasa albomarginata, chestnut, pearl barley, sanzukon) and underwent finger-pressure therapy, vacuum blood-purification therapy and others.

JANUARY 15, 1972

Visited an association for treatment with natural medicines.
Tried ozone therapy and acupuncture in addition to vacuum blood-purification therapy again for about one month. Not wanting to die, I had tried everything that might offer the slightest possibility

of stopping the growth of the tumor. Yet, I did not seem to have the slightest hope of recovering. My body was being eaten away inch by inch by a hideous growth and I had reached the stage where I thought that suicide might be a wiser choice.

FEBRUARY 3, 1972

I visited the Organic Germanium Clinic. Upon obtaining my case history in detail, they began administering a daily dose of 120 ml of water solution of organic germanium and of 200 mg of organic germanium powder.

MARCH 4, 1972

Dr. Asai of the Organic Germanium Clinic stressed the importance of the patient's own will to cure himself and suggested that I might seek a source of strong will power in religion. Thus, I joined the adherents of Temple Shinnyoen of the Shingon Esoteric School of Buddhism.

APRIL 20, 1972

The priest at Temple Shinnyoen predicted that I would have to remove the tumor.

MAY 1, 1972

The doctors at the Germanium Clinic diagnosed that lack of growth of the tumor indicated the arresting of activities of malignant cells. Destruction of the malignant cells by radiation was attempted. For reducing the harmful effect of radiation, a large dose of 1,000 mg of the germanium compound was administered.

JUNE 1, 1972

I began undergoing cobalt radiation treatment at Hospital K.

JULY 24, 1972

After a total of 47 administrations of cobalt radiation continuously, except for four days in between, I sustained no weakening in physical strength and my growing appetite surprised the doctor in charge.

The cobalt radiation treatment hardly caused changes in the blood data as shown in the subjoined table, except for the white blood cells and platelet counts that were at a near critical level. (These returned to normal 10 days after the radiation treatment was completed).

Blood Data Before and After Cobalt Radiation

	July 17	July 24 (After 47th radiation)
White blood cells	3,100	3,000
Red blood cells	507	513
Blood platelets	10.2	9.6
T.P.	7.4	7.4
A/G	1.5	1.55
GOT	37	35
GPT	28	30

AUGUST 8, 1972

Angiograms were taken. The angiographic examination began by local anaesthesia at 1 o'clock in the afternoon. I underwent a similar examination two years ago, and it was an agonizing experience.

I prayed, and I felt as though I were walking towards a path that led towards what seemed like a rising sun, but its rays were not glaring.

While I continued, I did not feel the slightest pain and I was filled with the satisfaction of having had a sound sleep in the morning. I heard only the whispering of the doctors and the mechanical sound of the apparatus.

Upon hearing the noises of photographing, I was told that the examination was over. During these two hours I felt no pain.

SEPTEMBER 3, 1972

Before undergoing the excision operation of the tumor, I went to the Temple Shinnyoen where I received the last message: "Buddha will provide protection only to those who leave their fate entirely to him."

SEPTEMBER 4, 1972

The operation was performed as scheduled. The four members of my family and the mother of Priest Fukuda of the Temple Shinnyoen and I prayed for the success of the operation before entering the operating room at 09:00 a.m. The operation lasted for 5 hours and 30 minutes to remove the cartilage tumor which weighed about two kilograms, requiring blood transfusion of 3,000 ml. I was returned to the ward at 14:00 p.m.

My father and my wife who were with me when I was operated on two years ago were surprised to see the marked difference between the color of my face after this operation and that after the previous operation. I looked so much better this time. When I came to, I did not feel the pain expected after a major operation of this sort.

The surgeon who performed the operation also told me that the operation could be carried out far more smoothly than the previous one.

On the third day I could eat ordinary food, and on the fourth day after operation I began to get up and walk about. On the 10th day the stitches were removed. The feared festering did not occur, nor was serum hepatitis caused despite the huge blood transfusion. My recovery was very quick.

SEPTEMBER 22, 1972

On the 18th day I was allowed to leave the hospital with the surgeon's assurance that I was on the road toward recovery.

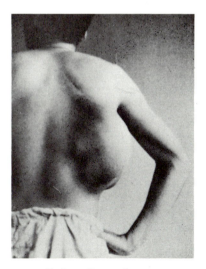
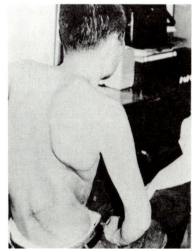

Before Operation　　　　　　After Operation
Cartilage Tumor

Three years ago when I was able to work in the field as a farmer, I used to complain of anything in the way. When it rained, I grumbled about the delay in my work because of the rain. When it shone, I complained about the heat, and when it was windy, I grumbled that it was too cold. If the day's turnover was small, I scolded the members of my family that they ought to work harder.

Now I live every day filled with joy and gratitude though I have no income. This life of gratitude I owe to Dr. Asai and all those who have guided and helped me, and I wish to thank each one of them.

6. My Struggle with Cancer of the Larynx

Dawn approaches. The clock hands point to four. I am not sleepy but I try my best to go to sleep.

The cigarette stubs piled high in the ashtray as I persisted and did 20 pages of manuscript for the day. Then, indulging in self-satisfaction, I rinsed out my mouth at the sink, and gargled with sodium bicarbonate in hot water.

When I write, I smoke. Then, before going to bed, I must wash out my throat with a soda solution. Finally, I take a good drink of germanium dissolved in water, and freed from the fear of cancer, I crawl into bed. However, this night when I gargled, it seemed as if something was stuck in my throat, and I discovered that it was difficult to raise my voice. Since I was feeling very drowsy I went to bed. In the morning when I awoke, I tried my voice and found that I was quite hoarse. I thought I had probably caught cold, but the hoarseness did not improve. I tried to sing a familiar song but the higher notes were no good and I did not feel like singing.

I was not conscious of anything wrong with my body, but for the last eight months I had been writing on my manuscript late every night, and became weary for I was not used to such activity. I was most anxious to finish so I could leave Tokyo during the hot, muggy, rainy season. I felt sure that I would be my old self again, and be over my hoarseness.

I gave my manuscript to the publisher, and flew to my mountain retreat shortly after the middle of July.

In early September I was scheduled to attend a World Congress on Natural Medicine in the city of Aix-en-Provence in France, and give a lecture under the title "The Efficacy of Treatment with Germanium, particularly as it relates to Cancer." However, before that I would have to do something about my voice, so I sent to a local drugist, and bought every kind of throat medicine he had. Of course, I continued taking germanium as well, but there was no sign of improvement. Then, there was a vast amount of ear wax in both ears and it became difficult to hear, but my appetite was good, I slept well, and during the day walked in my garden in good spirits, feeling sure that I would soon be well.

On September 8th we flew to France.

The content of the meeting and my impression of it, though of importance do not need to be detailed at this juncture. Suffice it to say that I was pleased to be able to continue my talk for more than twenty minutes even though my throat was so bad, and I was amazed by the rapidity with which those in attendance comprehended the presentation on germanium. After the conference we went to Germany where two of our children live.

When my son heard my voice he said, with eyebrows raised, "Early tomorrow morning you are to go to the hospital with me."

I answered him light-heartedly, "Don't worry about me, but I'll go with you as I'd like to see your hospital."

Through my son's introduction, it was arranged for me to be examined by Prof. Ronninghof, chief of the ear, nose, and throat department. He took my tongue between his fingers, pulled it out and looked into my throat, let out a shocked gasp, and turning to my son exclaimed, "How is this man still alive today? He has a polyp as big as my thumb in his windpipe, and could have died from asphyxiation."

My son was more excited than I. I had understood the Professor's German all right, but I could recall no difficulty in breathing, I felt very good physically so I was not greatly disturbed.

With the doctor's diagnosis, and my son's insistence, the next day I went into surgery, and had the polyp removed. Even when traveling I had not neglected to take my germanium, and especially in view of such an operation, I took an extra large dose.

When I came to after surgery, I felt no pain at all, but rather as though I had awakened from a deep sleep, fully refreshed. I got up, dressed myself, and took a taxi to my son's home. In the evening, three days later, my son, with a very grave face said, "As a result of the cellular examination of that polyp, they want to operate again just to make sure." He spoke as though he were hiding something.

I replied, "If cancer is confirmed, then I'll have surgery, but if not, then I prefer to return to Japan and be treated there."

My son, with his mind seemingly made up, explained "As a result of the cellular examination, it has been determined that a squamous cell carcinoma with high metastasizing tendency surrounds the vocal cords with cancerous cells. When the polyp was removed, some parts remained after surgery, and these must not be left. They will have to open up from the outside, and thoroughly cut away what surrounded the polyp that was removed. If the cancer spreads, they say you have not over two years to live."

My son knew that this would be a mental shock to me, but he did not beat around the bush. But instead of being shocked, I felt rather that this would be a good opportunity to prove germanium, and in high spirits I assured him, "Don't worry, I'll use germanium and cure myself."

The next morning I reluctantly entered the hospital for a second operation.

Just as the previous time, I awoke as from a good sleep, and wondered if after all I had really been operated on for throat cancer. But I felt the gauze around my neck and accepted the fact of the operation. At this time I recalled that a physician in Japan had told me of giving organic germanium to his patients a week before surgery who would then experience little discomfort and an early recovery.

There on my hospital bed I did some thinking. Unlike the temporary hocus pocus of traditional allopathic medicine, the effectiveness of germanium shows up in healing through the operation of elemental processes within man himself. In the different diseases, even cancer, there is no need to fear, and I developed the three conditions for the healing of cancer which have since brought hope for healing to those afflicted. Indeed, these conditions apply to all those undergoing organic germanium treatment for any disease. Briefly, there must be a deep conviction that one can surely heal himself with power he possesses. Secondly, diet is of the utmost importance; one's food must be planned so as to keep the blood from becoming acid. When the acid-base balance in the blood breaks down, the blood becomes acidic, and the oxygen in the hemoglobin of the red corpuscles loses its power. The capacity of the hemoglobin in the red blood cells to carry oxygen is diminished, and this brings about an oxygen deficiency in the body. Thirdly, oxygen deficiency in the body must be prevented. These conditions were set forth in greater detail in the introduction.

Late in life Dr. Hideyo Noguchi put forth the theory of one cause for all disease by declaring that all sickness originates from a single source, and from this developed the concept of one medicine for all ills. That single source was declared to be oxygen deficiency, a far-sighted view which can only be held in the highest esteem. The doctor worked on many experiments in an effort to find substances such as colloidal platinum and others that would produce oxygen in the body, but he died without seeing success from his efforts. If only he could have lived to see that the taking of organic germanium supplies the body with a considerable amount of oxygen through the blood, what joy he would have known!

I have always urged cancer patients to put complete confidence in my germanium, and with a simple desire on my part to save those suffering from cancer, I have enunciated these conditions. This may sound ideological or like self-importance on my part. Of course, there have been actual cases where cancer has been cured, and where the suffering from cancer has been alleviated, but these are not subjective conclusions on my part.

I myself have had cancer and since I have overcome it so beautifully with germanium as my weapon, I can provide genuine proof, for I have tested it on my own body, and everything I say has a powerful basis. This is bound to have great influence on all with whom I come in contact.

Such joyous thoughts must have shone on my face although I was not conscious of it. The surgeon said to my son, "I have been dealing with cancer patients for a long time, but your father is the first one I have ever seen to smile on learning that he had cancer. Perhaps this is the end."

On the fourth day after my surgery, I left the hospital, and went to my son's home, and on the fifth day, my wife and I took a plane bound for Tokyo.

I rested at home for a couple of months, but my neighbors who knew of my illness amazed me with all their concern on my behalf. As far as I was concerned both physically and emotionally, I firmly believed I had been completely freed from cancer. Intuitively people seemed to think that once a man developed cancer he was seized by the god of death.

My son in Germany became worried about me and urged me to have an examination in Japan, and also to take radiation therapy. Added to this was the concern of all the people around me. So I went to Keio University hospital from which my son had graduated, and had an examination by Dr. S., ear, nose, and throat specialist. He made several bioscopic examinations from my throat, and in the final diagnosis declared that there was no trace of cancer cells and hence no need for radiation.

Two and a half years have passed since my operation in Germany. I take 3 g of germanium daily, follow a well-regulated life regimen, am careful to avoid overwork, and abstain from tobacco strictly. My body tone is better than ever before, and I have gained 7 kg in weight.

I may have lost my beautiful voice, but I can savor the joy of telling people that cancer is not frightful, and of saving people from the suffering of a malignant disease.

7. Germanium and Leukemia

Late one night I was called on abruptly by a company employee. From his story I learned that his five-year-old son was in a government hospital with myelogenous leukemia. The doctor had said the case was hopeless, and because of various injections and medications, the boy's face was full of blisters, and his whole body covered with a rash. He had scratched himself till the skin was broken and bleeding, and there were openings on his sides from which the pus was discharging.

It was such a wretched condition that it made my body shiver just to hear about it. I told him to come early the next morning bringing the hospital's medical certificate with him, and sent him home.

I talked with the doctor at the Organic Germanium Clinic, instructing him to give the boy 2 g in solution each day, and since the man was financially embarassed, to cut the cost in half at least. Five days later the wife came and reported that the child's condition had improved astonishingly. The child had hated the quantity of medicine the doctor had prescribed at the hospital and had refused to take it. They had thrown out the medicine but there was nothing they could do about the injections. The child liked the germanium, however, and called it his "Water of Life."

According to later reports, the child began feeling very well, and was permitted to spend three days at home at the New Year. For the first time in months the family of four were all together and had a very happy New Year's day. During that time, he drank his "Water of Life" freely, ate heartily, and no one would have thought that he had been gravely ill. It is no wonder that he was so fretful about returning to the hospital.

The hospital pressed urgently for his return. Six days after returning to the hospital, the boy died. The couple came to my office three days afterward to express their appreciation to me. They wept as they told me how the child had taken the germanium, saying over and over "This is the water of life," as he did so.

When he died, they told me, there was a smile on his face, and no trace of suffering. His body warmth remained till the following morning.

Mr. F., an employee in the managerial department of a big company came to me with a letter of introduction. His eldest daughter, 9 years of age, had been diagnosed at the Tokyo University hospital as having myelogenous leukemia, and was waiting for a bed to open in the hospital. I told the father he must follow my instructions and his daughter would surely survive her "incurable" leukemia.

"First of all, you parents must show strong conviction that she will be healed. Number two, you must be careful of her diet to keep her body from acidity. Finally, you must give her large doses of germanium regularly."

Mr. F. listened thoughtfully to what I said, then straightening up slowly, replied, "Dr. Asai, I can only say yes, by all means! The doctor says she has only a year to live. Please help us."

I told him to get the hospital diagnosis and go to my clinic at once, have a consultation with the doctor, and start treatment with germanium. I also made contact with the clinic.

Three years have now passed, and the girl is in first year of middle school, perfectly healthy, and attending school in good spirits. She continues to take my germanium faithfully.

I received a letter from a Mr. O. studying art in Vienna, who told me that his nine-year-old daughter had been diagnosed at the Tokyo University hospital as having a bone tumor in the right arm. He asked that I contact his wife and advise her.

For some unknown reason his nine-year-old daughter had suddenly developed severe pain in her right arm. As a result of an examination she was found to have a virulent bone tumor, and they proposed cutting out a part of the bone and making a transplant from a portion of bone from the mother's hip bone.

As I always do, I told her that the healing of her daughter was in her hands and not that of the doctor's. First of all she must stay calm for the child's sake. She must not be agitated, or be nervous, but surround the girl with an atmosphere of tranquility that would give her confidence.

She must be extremely careful of the girl's diet to keep her body from becoming acid. She must avoid all medications, and use only an ample amount of germanium.

This was exactly the same method as I gave in the previous examples, and good results depended entirely on her carrying out all the instructions to the letter.

Mrs. O. accepted all my remarks sincerely, and returned home.

The girl continued having monthly examinations, but there was no more talk about an operation, and she continued attending school with no hindrances. She did not take part in the physical exercises or the school competitions, or other violent activities, but otherwise has continued for three years living a normal, healthy life.

Case report (Leukemia, male, 12 years old): Diagnosed as suffering from leukemia at a hospital, the patient underwent chemotherapy, but no relief was obtained from such symptoms as fever, fatigue and bleeding gums. At our clinic, a dose of 500 mg of water solution of the organic germanium compound was administered, and on the 3rd day his temperature returned to normal and stayed there all month.

The patient regained enough strength to go to school again. Two months later, the blood count at the hospital where he received the initial information of his disease revealed no abnormality.

Before we could produce the organic germanium compound, we prepared a germanium salt solution and injected it into an albino rat whose hematogenic tissues of the bone marrow had been destroyed by irradiation of radioactive rays. The hematogenic tissues were found restored in the marrow when dissected about three weeks later. This experiment was presented at a meeting of the Radiological Society.

Germanium proved to be particularly effective in treating leukemia among children, and while in many cases the disease could be arrested, just as many children entirely recovered.

8. Death of a Widow

With the witness of people who have been saved by my germanium, and with the letters of gratitude piling in veritable mountains, if I should try to write them all it would not only become stale remarks, but would sound like a cheap publication, and I have no urge for that.

Cancer is considered a fatal disease and it has come to the point where of late the medical world simply throws up its hands when faced with the incurable. Thus many people, grasping at a straw, come inquiring at my Organic Germanium Clinic. Sadly enough, most of those who do come are in the last stages of the illness.

Nearly all of those who come have not been told by their doctors that they have cancer, but the doctor's "sentence of death" has reached their relatives, and with the hope of escaping death, they come with their earnest appeals.

One fine autumn afternoon, three middle-aged women came to visit me. The purpose had to do with the sickness of one of them, a lady around fifty years of age. The other two were looking after her. She had been to my Organic Germanium Clinic, and the doctor had prescribed germanium following his examination, but apparently she wanted to make doubly sure and had come to see me.

I immediately phoned the clinic and inquired as to the nature of the illness. They informed me that she had cancer of the liver which had spread to the peritoneum, and there was an accumulation of abdominal fluid. She had gone to the K hospital but they could do nothing for her.

I always tell the sick that it is they who must do the healing and not the doctors or medicine. To illustrate, I explained to the woman thus: "Let's say this wristwatch has stopped running. I am the one who is inconvenienced and no one else has any concern. I plead with the watch to start running but it has no effect. But then if I have a little screw driver, I fix the watch. It is the same way with sickness. You yourself must do the healing, and for that you need a tool. That tool is oxygen, occurring and active in your body, and germanium produces it within you."

Then, I painstakingly explained to her how she must exercise extreme care with her diet in order to preserve the acid-base balance in the blood, and how she must develop peace of mind, and not worry about anything. My visitor seemed relieved and returned to the K hospital where she was a patient.

In a previous book, I wrote as follows: "It is considered taboo for an amateur to say anything about cancer. All I can say then is that cancer differs from diseases in general, or that it is a fate man is destined to bear, I do not say that germanium is a symptomatic treatment for cancer. What I do emphasize is that it frees man from the hands of the devil."

One morning six days later, I received a phone call from one of the attendants of that lady who told me that after taking germanium, the abdominal fluid was relieved, her body condition eased greatly, and her doctor after consultation told her to return home for recuperation. The lady apparently wanted to see me and had expressed her desire for me to go to her home.

I was led into a beautiful, spacious room, and there on a bed lay the widowed lady. I had no knowledge of her wealth and the inheritancy involved, but I could not help guessing from her statements that her attachment to that inheritance together with her anxiety over it had contributed largely to her illness, and had deprived her of an important element in the healing of her disease. When I learned that the doctor was coming every day to give her an anticancer injection, I was completely discouraged.

During the next 20 days I maintained her supply of germanium.

Once more I went to her home in answer to an urgent telephone call. From her sick bed she greeted me with these words, "Dr. Asai, my husband is calling me from heaven, saying Come, come soon. I, too, want to go to him at once. I want you to hear this song. Dr. Asai, you have been a great help to me, and I can never forget your kindness. In parting, I want to give you this record I have made. Please listen to it with me now."

These are the words I listened to from the stereo close by:

> Rose, Oh beautiful rose,
> Pure and fragrant upon the earth.
> You are the gift I offer;
> Reflecting heaven's splendor,
> You are the gift I offer.

Her complexion was good, and instead of showing any suffering, her face wore a smile that gave her a celestial appearance. As I left I laid my right hand on her brow and said to myself, "This is best, rest in peace."

From the family I learned that she had passed away that night as one peacefully dropping off to sleep. They reported that her body had remained warm till the afternoon of the next day and had not grown rigid. The family had folded her hands over her bosom and her form was so beautiful and so angel-like that they found themselves pressing their palms together in an attitude of veneration. From a later conversation, I learned that following cremation, when the cremation tray was withdrawn from the furnace, the bones in it were the color of the *sakuragai* (the Tellina, or literally cherry shell), and retained their original shape. The folk had actually felt like preserving them instead of placing them in the burial urn.

When people die of cancer, not only does the agony of death usually remain on their face, but it is said that even after cremation, the traces of cancer invasion can be clearly detected in the bones. One wonders if this is the result of the final struggle with the demon death that drains all strength when life ebbs out in utter exhaustion. However, germanium performs the glorious role of knocking out this demon, driving him away and then peacefully leading the soul to the feet of God.

9. Death of a Maiden

The god of death, if he has an opening, mercilessly attacks even the young, and it is absolutely futile to try to combat him with ordinary methods.

Strangely enough, a girl of 18 or 19 years with an incurable brain tumor provides such as example. The January 20, 1968 issue of the Japan Economic newspaper, carried an article of mine under the title, "A 20-year obsession with germanium," in which I wrote of the therapeutic effectiveness of germanium.

The next morning an elderly gentleman I took to be about 60 years of age, called on me. He had come to see me after learning my address from the newspaper. "Dr. Asai," he said, "My 19-year-old daughter is suffering from a brain tumor, and the doctors have given up. I want you to help her with germanium."

I questioned him further and learned that two years earlier, she had suffered from severe headaches, and he had taken her to the neurosurgical department of the Tokyo University hospital for an examination. This resulted in a diagnosis of brain tumor, and she had undergone surgery and returned home. They had told him that she had no more than two years to live.

After two years there was a relapse and she was taken to the hospital again. The attending doctor declared that there was nothing to do but operate, but there was no assurance she would live through the operation. Since she was still alive, the father chose to take her home. The headaches grew increasingly worse, and he could not stand to see her suffer. As a parent myself, I could easily understand how this father could not bear the thought of his daughter dying at the very threshold of adulthood. More than that, the thought of this innocent, pure maiden being so suddenly attacked by the god of death filled me with rage, and I was moved with zeal to join battle with him at once.

I gave the father a 0.2% solution of my synthesized organic germanium and told him she should drink 40 ml, and thereafter take the same amount before breakfast, dinner, and supper, three times each day. I told him that for germanium to exert its force, her food intake should be regulated to avoid blood acidity. Then I told him to stop using all medicine prescribed by the hospital. I also pointed out how important it was to believe in the germanium. In the case of a child, the influence of the parents is extremely great, so they must deal with this matter in an attitude of prayer.

In his book, *Man, The Unkown*, Alexis Carrel makes a statement with which I whole-heartedly concur. He writes:

"...However, following the great scientific experiments of the 19th Century, this faith man has completely lost. Not only is the view widely held that there have been no miracles in the past, but that there is no possibility of any miracles being performed in the future. Just as the laws of thermodynamics make perpetual motion an impossibility, the laws of biological science recognize no miracles. This is the current attitude of biologists and doctors in general.

However, the facts we have gathered up to now do not support such an attitude. The most important facts show up in evidence collected in the medical bureau at Lourdes. Our general concept of the influence of prayer on diseased conditions results largely from the observation of almost instantaneous healing of such illnesses as tuberculosis of the bones, tubercular peritonitis, liver abcesses, osteitis, festering wounds, skin lesions (lupus,) and cancer.

The healing process differs but little with different individuals. Sometimes it is accompanied by intense suffering, then suddenly there surges a feeling of recovery from the illness. Then in a few seconds, or a few minutes, or at least in a few hours, the wounds close, the symptoms disappear, and the appetite returns. It cannot be doubted that the miraculous recovery is exceedingly more rapid than ordinary recovery from an illness.

The absolutely essential element in this is prayer. While this is true, it does not mean that the sick person himself does the praying nor that the sick person himself must hold certain religious convictions. It is enough if there is someone in an attitude of prayer at the sick person's side.

Such facts as these hold an extremely important meaning, and they reveal that in the relationship between the mind and the body, there is an element we do not know. They reveal to us objectively the consequence of the actions of the mind, something the hygienists, the doctors, the educators, and the sociologists have shown practically no intention of studying. We are standing at the doorway to a new world."

It was the evening of the following day when I received a telephone call from the father who had called on me the previous day and gone home with some germanium. "Dr. Asai," he said, "the headaches have left her like a bad dream, and her appetite has returned. Is it all right to feed her?"

"That's fine," I replied, "I'm happy to hear it. Avoid meat and acid-forming foods as far as possible, and give her *tofu* (bean curd), vegetables, with some vinegar, as well as sardines."

Three days later I prepared five 500 ml bottles of germanium solution and took them to the patient's home.

I have often gone in condolence to the sick beds of young people, who were usually suffering from cancer or severe rheumatism, and so often, when I entered, the atmosphere of the place, the light, the room arrangement, the odors, and the impressions I got from the people gave me sensations in my skin that cannot be described. Something like a dark, damp atmosphere seems to strike my forehead and cheeks, and I find it hard to breathe. Conditions in this house were the same.

I wanted to do anything I could save this girl from an incurable disease, so with a prayer in my heart I took her hand and earnestly explained the power of germanium. I dreamt of making this girl well, and then have her come and work for me as a symbol of the power of germanium.

The young girl took a remarkable turn for the better. She left her bed to sit in the sun on the verandah, and joined the family at the table at meal time. Folks around her naturally looked upon the results as miraculous, for it was something they could not have imagined up to a short time ago. I never failed to go each month to her home and take her germanium.

The young lass made every effort, even to the point of tears, to overcome her malady. Every time I looked at her, I grew exasperated as I wondered if there was not some way to speed up her recovery.

Thus that year passed, and the girl was able to greet New Year's Day of 1969. January 15 was to be Adults' Day for her that year. As I saw the other girls of her age in their gay clothes filling the streets and frolicking with their companions, I impulsively bought a red sweater and took it to her home. The mother met me at the door and said, "Since morning my daughter has not felt well, and has remained in bed. I'm glad you have come. Please try to cheer her up."

I went at once to her bedside, but why should she seem to be pouting when I came in, turn her face away, pretend to be sleeping, and not greet me at all? Perhaps she had a headache.

I told the mother of the Adults' Day celebrations, and leaving the sweater, I returned home. Ten days later, I felt somewhat disturbed and went to her home again.

That day she seemed to be in better spirits. She was sitting in a chair beside her bed, gazing into the corner of the room. She became conscious of my presence, and reached out and picked up from beside her bed, a package wrapped in paper, and without a word handed it to me. In it was a little basket daintily woven from colored straw. I took the basket from her hand and gazed at it for a while. I could not hold back the tears that filled my eyes.

Without doubt she had worked hard with her crippled hands and woven that basket just to make me happy. I could stand it no longer, and as I left the house I cried out in my heart, Mephisto, you demon who torments this sweet little girl, take away your hand. There are many others in the world you might make to suffer. Mephisto, get out and leave!

Although the girl had regained her vitality to that extent, by autumn of that year she was again confined to her bed. This was due to the sudden appearance of a lump on the back of her head with a swelling of the scalp.

From the father I learned that at the first operation, they found that the cancer cells had penetrated quite deeply and could not completely be removed. The opening in the spinal column for the spinal fluid was also clogged with cancer cells and a tube had been put in the spinal column so the fluid could flow. Such a medical procedure was nothing more than a phony makeshift, but present medical science seems to have no other course outside such a method.

Our present medical science is impotent against the evil spirit who lurks stealthily in the great world of nature, waiting for the opportunity to work mischief on humanity and cause them suffering. Based on my experience, organic germanium in large doses causes the cancer cells to break down and form into thick, darkred pus. This is due to the fact that cancer cells are protein and when they are broken down, they decay and indisputably they produce poisonous substances as a consequence. In some cases these are expelled from the body naturally, but in many cases they remain in the body. If such is the case, these putrified elements must be removed at once. In this way a patient in the last stages of stomach cancer was saved, and also a man with a cartilaginous tumor on his side as big as a watermelon was healed.

I was certain beyond the shadow of a doubt that the swelling on the back of the little girl's head was just such a thing.

I urged the father repeatedly to take her immediately to the neurosurgical department of the Tokyo University hospital for a consultation where she had been previously examined. The father stubbornly refused. Once a man gives way to unbelief, his whole nervous system builds up a negative reaction irrespective of logic.

Whether the father saw the surgeon's scalpel at the Tokyo University hospital as the devil's claw, or whether he thought that the doctor's treatment was not to save his precious daughter but rather to take her life, in spite of my earnest counsel he refused to the end to say yes.

In this instance I discover the fateful cause and effect of man's life.

I said to that stubborn father that what I urged did not mean an operation but only the removing of impurities from the body. I continued to press the matter but with him it was only futile.

I increased the dosage of germanium to the girl. It had already been tested thoroughly for toxicity and proved absolutely nontoxic. Moreover, I had tested it in my own body with up to 5 g in one day, and had her take over a period of time, 3 g per day, one before each meal.

The girl's condition while not good, still showed no particularly bad elements. With no signs of fluctuation, she remained on her sick bed for three years after beginning germanium treatment.

While germanium prevents illness from worsening into death, some day the sword may break or the arrows be spent. Still, this is only an observation on dillydallying, and on effectiveness in prolonging life, and has no relation whatsoever to recovery from illness.

Again I tried to convince that father but again I was unsuccessful. On the contrary he stopped germanium and began Chinese herbs, to my further consternation.

One day late in June as the end of the humid, rainy season drew near, I suddenly got a phone call from the girl's mother, telling me that in spite of all her efforts to live, the girl had died. While no one was watching she had passed away as though falling asleep.

Following the deathwatch I wrote in that day's journal, the little girl was by no means taken away by the god of death. God had called his beloved to his home to save her from suffering. As proof did her face not shine vividly, a smile play around her lips, and did she not look like one of heaven's maidens? The death of a loved one is so holy that one can only pray in silence.

When she was placed in the coffin with her face surrounded with flowers, in no way did it appear as the face of one dead. There was no trace of the suffering from that fateful disease. Her form as one unconscious in sleep, seemed like a princess from fairyland, or a sleeping nymph from the forest.

When placing her into the coffin, according to her mother, there was no rigidity in her body, and thinking of her again as a child, she had held her in her bosom. The body was still warm, and the mother said they hesitated to place the corpse in the coffin.

When they placed their hands in the bed where the girl had been it was still warm, and they were cheered by the thought that she had not died but had peacefully gone to heaven led by the hand of God.

After cremation, the remaining bones were of a dainty cherry shell color, and the Adam's apple in particular remained without crumbling. Those involved were astonished that the ashes could not be contained in the burial urn.

From inquiry, I learned that five days before her death, the girl had spat out a large amount of foul-smelling matter like thickened blood. This convinced me even more that I had not been wrong in my judgment.

10. Peaceful Death

A doctor friend of mine in Yokohama sent me the following report.

"I have been amazed at the effectiveness of germanium. I was asked to examine an inoperable patient in whom cancer, beginning in the lungs, had spread to the liver, the pancreas, and to all his organs.

He was a male about 50 years old and was in such pain that his loud cries disturbed the other patients, and he had to be given large quantities of morphine to induce sleep. Even this was insufficient, so they put him in a bed with wheels on it, and had moved him to the front of the morgue.

I had organic germanium with me and gave him successively five hypodermic injections of 40 mg in 2 ml ampules. I left ten more ampules with the nurses with instructions to continue giving them till the next morning, and returned home.

The next day I had a phone call from the hospital reporting that after the injections, the patient became energetic, was hungry, and asked for food.

I put germanium injection solution in my bag and hastened to the hospital. When I arrived, they were just ready to start administering a glucose solution by intravenous injection. I added germanium solution to the drip solution, and left 15 ampules for injection every two hours.

I did not go to the hospital after that but was informed by the hospital that the cyanosis, that is, the dark purple color of the face so characteristic of cancer patients, had changed to a living flesh color, his pain was gone, and he was in good spirits. In fact, he had suddenly wanted to make known his last will, and had asked that his family be called. His family arrived, and at great length he had given instructions as to what should be done after his death. Two days later, as if dropping off to sleep, he had died peacefully."

11. Concluding Remarks

Cancer is an incurable disease. There are various means of treating it, such as carcinostatic substances and radiotherapy, but it is undeniable that none of these treatments offers conclusive efficacy.

I would like to state that organic germanium is indispensable in treating cancer. It is needed not only for treating benign tumors but also for all obstinate diseases arising from malignant tumors. However, if the disorder is diagnosed as cancer, the earlier the administration of germanium the greater the effect. In any case, even a "wonder drug" will naturally be ineffective if the disease is in the terminal stage or the "cachexia" due to cancer has progressed too far.

What is most distressing in the case of cancer is the pain attending the terminal stage. Anodyne is usually injected continuously in an attempt to relieve the pain. Only organic germanium can relieve this pain resulting from terminal cancer. When organic germanium is injected into a patient with advanced cancer who can no longer take the drug orally, the pain and suffering miraculously subside.

To give a final example, there was a man aged 64 years, whose doctor had given him only six months to live with lung cancer. When this patient began to take organic germanium, he lived through the first six months, and though he caught a cold he lasted through one year. This man ultimately died after a year and seven months from an asthma spasm caused by an aggravated summer cold, but his death was painless.

I said earlier that it was difficult to make an objective assessment of the overall effect of germanium in the treatment of cancer. Cancer is a disease causing those afflicted mental and physical agonies far beyond those imaginable in any other disease. The majority of the patients who come to the Organic Germanium Clinic are in the last stages of their disease. They turn to us as a last resort. Mostly they are too weak to appear in person and are represented by a relative in a last desperate effort to help the afflicted escape imminent death.

Of the patients who are now being treated with germanium, most refuse to return to modern medicine, but remain at home and continue germanium treatment. One youth began germanium treatment after receiving notice from his hospital that his case was hopeless, and is now well. Many in worse conditions with only a day or two to live, have extended their lives three months, a year, two years, and in some cases even four years with germanium. Most of all, however, these people appreciated the relief from intense suffering brought by treatment with germanium. The unfortunate for whom it was too late to extend their lives passed away peacefully freed from the agonies associated with cancer.

Future Trend in Medical Treatment— Inducement of the Body's Natural Healing Power

The other day I had an interesting conversation with a friend now living comfortably in retirement. This friend had earlier been successfully treated with my organic germanium compound and had become a firm believer in its efficacy. For many years he had been suffering from ringing in the ears, and although various medical cures had been attempted, he had gained little relief. Treatment with organic gernium, however, completely healed his ailment, and furthermore, his general health showed a most remarkable improvement. In fact, one would hardly suspect that this healthy gentleman had already lived over 70 years. Borne out of a philanthropic spirit and on the basis of his own experience, he decided to use my organic germanium compound (without infringing on any pharmaceutical regulations) to help other people suffering from incurable diseases. Not surprisingly, he has been very successful in his efforts, much to the gratitude of a large number of people.

My friend had this to say: "Rather than being similar to modern pharmaceutical medicines, this organic germanium compound is more like one of the traditional Chinese medicinal herbs. I have used it to treat a number of different illnesses, and have found its healing effect to be more constitutional than allopathic—that is, it acts on the body as a whole rather than on any specific symptom.

"To put it more simply, your organic germanium cures diseases by inducing the body's own natural healing powers. I am convinced that by increasing the flow of oxygen, organic germanium stimulates latent deficiency in modern medicine.

As I read in his book of the healing powers of the miracle water of Lourdes, I thought instinctively of its striking similarity to my organic germanium.

Why is germanium so miraculously effective against disease?—the puzzle has not yet been solved, but the secret seems to lie in its molecular system. Organic germanium has a strong hydrogen-combining force due to the many unstable oxygen atoms in it. When there is an oxygen deficiency in the human system, the blood becomes acid and sickness results. However, organic germanium, because of its special tendency of hydrogen attachment, unites with the hydrogen which is then thrown off from the body, and the oxygen that remains does its effective work in the cells. This may clarify somewhat the puzzle of the water of Lourdes and the holy water of *Yamabuki* which have engendered faith in so many people. Indeed, it seems that those who are spiritually motivated are those that have benefited the most from organic germanium compound.

2. Water of Lourdes

In the Pyrenees on the French-Spanish border, there is a small village named Lourdes with a population of about 10,000. Numerous hotels, boarding houses and inns are clustered all over town and around its famous cathedral and its even more famous vicinity, accommodating guests from all over the world. By far the largest contingent of these people are comprised by the ailing who seek a cure with the help of the healing waters gushing out of the rock on which the cathedral is built.

The August 9, 1971, issue of the *Newsweek* carried the following story:

"A three-year-old girl contracted kidney cancer. One of the kidneys was excised, but the cancer spread to the cranial bone. She became emaciated, her hair had fallen out and her skin had turned yellow. Her whole system was affected by cancer and the doctors had given up her case as hopeless.

As a last resort, the parents sat her in a wheel-chair and went to

Lourdes, where the cancer-stricken girl was dipped in the sacred water of which she also drank. No sign of improvement appeared, and the discouraged parents brought their daughter back to Glasgow, Scotland, to let her die at home.

On the morning of the third day after their return, the girl suddenly sat up in bed and asking for an orange she began eating it. From then on her condition began to improve and several days later, the tumor disappeared and she was once again a healthy girl."

This story was accompanied by a photograph showing the girl in good spirits. This even created a major sensation in the medical circles of Scotland, and the fame of the miraculous water of Lourdes spread widely.

I have analysed some of the "miracle water" and found that it contains a relatively high amount of germanium. It must be said that I have no information as to what other compounds are contained in the Lourdes water, but in comparison with other waters the amount of germanium was far greater.

In *Man, the Unknown*, Dr. Alexis Carrel writes:

"Man enchanted by the remarkable progress in the sciences of lifeless matter (such as physics and chemistry) has not realized that the body and mind of man are governed by laws as precise as those

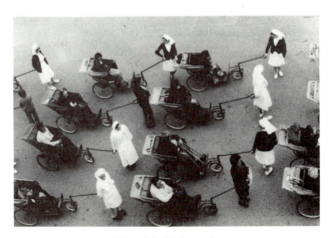

The sick in Lourdes

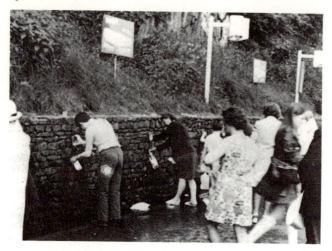

People drinking the Water of Lourdes.

governing the stars, and yet they are far more mysterious; moreover, man does not know that he is on the verge of danger as soon as he violates these laws."

In the same book he says, "I have attempted to make clear the fact that things still unknown remain to be solved, but that there are things that are entirely beyond the range of human knowledge." Organic germanium is a substance directly bound up in some way with life, and this discovery has impelled me into the mysterious world within nature that is beyond the wisdom of man.

3. Yamabuki-no-Omizu (Mountain Rose Spring)

I have dwelled upon the water of Lourdes since it has shown miraculous efficacy on cancer and other severe diseases and in this respect bears a strong resemblance to the action of germanium compound that I developed.

Guided by the distinct germanium line traced on the chart recorded by the atomic absorption meter when analysing the Lourdes water, and assuming that there is also a spring in Japan which is

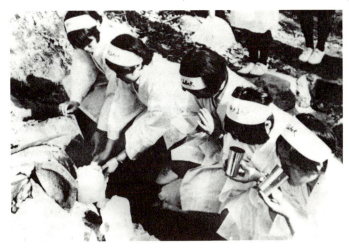

Shintoist Followers Drinking "Yamabuki no Omizu" from an underground spring deep in the mountains of Northern Japan

similar to the spring of Lourdes, I began investigating wonder-working waters such as hot spring waters popularly believed to be a cure for diseases. I finally came across a spring called *Yamabuki-no-Omizu* (Mountain Rose Spring) which particularly attracted my attention. It is located on a mountain on the northern tip of the Island of Honshu. The spring belongs to a mountain retreat of a Shintoist sect, its followers having been reported cured of obstinate diseases by drinking the water from this spring.

Unlike the tourist atmosphere in Lourdes, there was a simple, wooden chapel and prayer hall. About five kilometers further up the mountain, stood a small shrine surrounded by large trees. Aside the shrine gushed out "Yamabuki-no-Omizu" which was led through a bamboo pipe to facilitate drinking.

I picked up a wooden ladle lying nearby and scooped up a mouthful of water, which I kept in my mouth and swallowed in sips. It was cold and had a pure fresh taste. I brought a bottle of this water back to Tokyo for analysis. As with the water taken from Lourdes, the water from this spring indicated a clear line of germanium.

In the area covering the three northernmost prefectures of Honshu, mineral veins of metamorphic rock (this is a high pressure, thermal water-type ore, commonly called black ore) are widely distributed. In addition to a high iron content, the ore contains gold, silver, copper and zinc. Germanium has been extracted mainly from slag obtained by smelting copper or zinc ore.

On analyzing the black ore, my expectation that it surely contained germanium was confirmed. Various questions arose concerning the water called *Yamabuki-no-Omizu*: How did the germanium in the ore get into the underground stream, and how could the inorganic germanium in the ore change into organic germanium content in the water?

During the course of my research in the past, I once took up the problem as to why organic sulphur is contained in coal. Sulphur in coal presents problems when it comes to the stage of steel manufacture as it causes the quality of the steel to deteriorate, in addition it produces toxic sulfurous acid gas when burned. Inorganic sulphur can be removed from coal through coal dressing, but there are no ways of removing organic sulphur in coal.

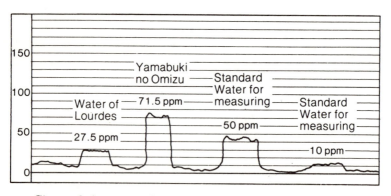

Chart of the germanium contents in the *Water of Lourdes* and *Yamabuki no Omizu* as measured on atomic absorption photometer.
(Note: Water taken from Lourdes was concentrated twice and *Yamabuki no Omizu* three times).

During my search for an explanation of the cause that changes inorganic sulphur into its organic form, I conducted a series of experiments, through which at last I found the answer that this metamorphosis is the work of certain bacteria. Using a highly magnifying microscope on samples taken from sulphur springs the existence of sulphur-eating bacteria could be confirmed.

In *Kagaku* (Chemistry) Vol. 28 No. 3, a scientific magazine published by Iwanami Publishers, I read a report that Prof. Voronkov who heads a chemical laboratory in Soviet Russia, maintained at the Third International Conference on Organic Silicon Chemistry that silicon bacteria exist and the microbes synthesize not only Si-O-C or Si-N-C combinations but also Si-C combination in the body.

Both silicon and germanium are typical semiconductors and widely distributed on the earth, and are considered to have played an important role in the origin of life. Thus the existence of germanium bacteria is naturally conceivable, and it stands to reason that as with silicon bacteria, these bacteria have the ability of turning the inorganic into the organic form, thus relating it with the life cycle.

With all the aforementioned as a base I have come to the conclusion that it is germanium that is the source of the miracle brought by the Water of Lourdes and the *Yamabuki-no-Omizu*.

4. Germanium Bathing

Whilst discussing the "miracle" waters perhaps it would not be inappropriate at this point to mention the germanium bath. This is the latest development in the administration of germanium which, as I have mentioned previously, is given orally, by injection, and may be applied directly to the affected area.

It goes without saying that nothing is more important to body improvement than a good metabolism. Yet, strangely enough, after much sweating from a germanium bath, people come out with no feeling of exhaustion at all.

Artist Eisetsu Shiratori, who made use of the bath, reported his experience as follows: "I was very tired when I arrived yesterday, and even though I stayed up late visiting, I slept soundly last night, and not only had my weariness disappeared, but I felt invigorated. This is the first time I have had such an experience. This morning I felt a strong urge to get back to work. Thank you for the wonderful bath." It was amazing to see how pleased he was.

There are many examples like this. One old man who had suffered from neuralgia for many years found relief, and came back every third day. A middle-aged woman who had had stubborn constipation of eight years rejoiced when the trouble left her as if it had been a bad dream.

Mr. Yanagizawa's report included the following:
1. After two or three minutes in the bath, the body became covered with large drops of perspiration.
2. After the bath, the whole body continued to glow with warmth.
3. After two or three times in the bath, leg and hip pains all but disappeared and the persons could walk with ease.
4. People with persistent constipation completely recovered, and were able to have regular and normal bowel movements.
5. People developed good appetites and could hardly wait for mealtime, and then they ate heartily.
6. Individuals with low blood pressure or poor circulation, once their bodies had been warmed, had no trouble with insomnia or with body chilling, and they had no distress when they got up in the morning.
7. A fat woman, from Aichi Prefecture, whose feet had turned purple in the forepart, found them light again after two or three times in the bath and was able to walk without trouble.
8. A woman secretary from Tokyo, after treatment at Kurbad returned home with a happy face free from her nervous condition and from the weariness of travel.

5. Religion, Divination and Germanium

I often find myself thinking about the wisdom of the people of ancient times. The *Eki*, or the Chinese art of divination, is said to have been developed through 5,000 years. It is an immense collection of acquired wisdom by the ancient people. As one master of this art of divination said, divination was originally meant to clarify the movements of the stars, the sun and the moon, the formation of heaven and earth, and the development process of human intellect, thereby explaining in great detail the creation and evolution of life including human beings. In short, it is a condensed form of description of nature.

This art defines everything related to the creation and evolution of the human world in a theory of dividing everything into the positive and the negative. Based on this theory, it divines the progress of the heaven, earth and man which comprise the universe. Since food for survival of man is related to the creation and evolution of human beings, food is an important field of the art of divination, on which the traditional Chinese medicine is based and the Oriental medicine has been developed.

A certain cycle of phenomena in nature that is widely known may be considered to be a kind of transmigration. Metallic elements in the soil are absorbed by plants, thereby contributing to the growth of these plants, while animals take metallic elements into their bodies by eating these plants. Within the body, inorganic metallic elements are turned organic. These elements are eventually returned to the soil through discharge or death. It is conceivable that certain elements including germanium contribute to the growth of life following the orbit of transmigration in nature. If we introduce this orbit of transmigration of germanium into our living system, we can avoid the contraction of even such diseases as cancer and maintain health in conformity with the law of nature. This has been my train of thought.

Germanium is indispensable to transistors. If this useful element in the forefront of the electronics industry plays an important role in the maintenance of health, it is clearly to be considered providential. I once published these thoughts in a newspaper article, and obtained surprising repercussions from readers. My telephone rang from early morning till late at night, and scores of visitors came to see me. Letters I received from all over the country were too numerous to answer. Most of those who contacted me wished to consult me about their ailments and obstinate diseases. What impressed me most then was lack of confidence among so many people in modern medicine and their ignorance regarding the close relationship between food and health.

Another surprise was the number of prominent persons from religious and divination circles who called me on account of that article. These people showed an inordinate interest in germanium. Those in the religious circles appeared mostly to be of the opinion that germanium will serve greatly as an aid in curing spiritual and physical troubles through faith in God or Buddha. Most of those engaged in divination welcomed the news of germanium, saying that they had long expected the emergence of germanium as the substance for saving mankind.

I asked several of them to divine the number 32 which is the atomic number of germanium. All agreed that "the substance is the origin of all creatures and substances and forms the center of all things in the universe and performs miracles." The fact that all the diviners told me the same with only a slight difference in wording gave me quite a thrill. I talked with these people about the fortunes of germanium. In short, they expounded the law of a world that is impossible for men to know. I surmised that they meant to say man must not disregard or defy this law.

From this, I concluded with conviction that germanium is a four-dimensional substance directly connected with life and is essentially different from conventional pharmaceuticals.

I have received countless letters of appreciation from people cured of their diseases through germanium therapy. These letters represent case histories of various obstinate diseases. Invariably the writers of these letters urged me to relieve others who are suffering from similar diseases by making this organic germanium compound available for them as soon as possible. These words moved me deeply and made me realize that man is good at heart after all in spite of this callous world.

There is always something special in the happiness one feels upon recovery from disease, which makes it essentially different from

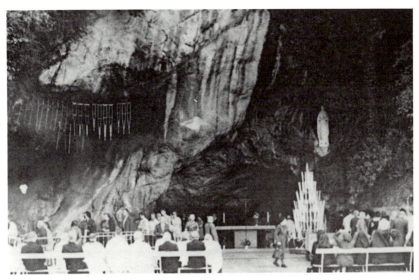

The sick visiting Lourdes offer prayers here before drinking the miracle water.

other pleasures. The voices of these people strike a particularly responsive cord in our hearts. Nevertheless, countless people suffering from obstinate diseases still do not have access to the organic germanium compound I have discovered. Men do not even know of its existence. Some fail to understand its amazing efficacy. All those who have been cured with germanium express their deep graditude for their encounter with the organic germanium compound therapy, which makes me all the more eager that everyone should utilize this therapy in the future. As I have repeatedly stressed, the germanium therapy is essentially different from mere symptomatic treatments; it is closely related to the essential characteristics of man. The difference may be likened to the difference between a brass band playing a march and an orchestra playing a symphony. In other words, the germanium therapy not only depends on the increased oxygen supply to the body cells but on something that cannot be fully explained merely in the usual scientific terms.

The sick visiting the spring of Lourdes always attend a solemn mass and offer their fervent prayers before drinking the miracle water. Those who drink *Yamabuki-no-Omizu* are pious believers with an ardent faith in Shintoism. I do believe that something unknown and impossible to know exists to give the miracle water the healing power.

When the 67 elements indispensable for living things are arranged in a single horizontal row in the order of the atomic numbers, beginning with hydrogen, germanium is located at the 32nd position or just in the middle of the row. This atom concurrently has the properties of positive and negative ions. In the Chinese art of divination, everything in the universe is considered to be governed by *ki* made up by the positive and the negative. I am inclined to think that germanium is precisely something that corresponds to this "ki" (prana). Chinese medicine is said to be established on the concept of *ki*, and Chinese physiology maintains that there are two circulation systems in the human body, and there are two substances that circulate in these systems: "intangible *ki*" and "tangible blood." The blood circulates in blood vessels and the *ki* circulates in channels of *ki* thoughout the body.

A considerable number of phenomena confirmed through the long process of history by the Oriental medicine remain inexplicable in terms of the present level of development in science.

Future Trend in Medical Treatment—Inducement of the Body's Natural Healing Power

The other day I had an interesting conversation with a friend now living comfortably in retirement. This friend had earlier been successfully treated with my organic germanium compound and had become a firm believer in its efficacy. For many years he had been suffering from ringing in the ears, and although various medical cures had been attempted, he had gained little relief. Treatment with organic gernium, however, completely healed his ailment, and furthermore, his general health showed a most remarkable improvement. In fact, one would hardly suspect that this healthy gentleman had already lived over 70 years. Borne out of a philanthropic spirit and on the basis of his own experience, he decided to use my organic germanium compound (without infringing on any pharmaceutical regulations) to help other people suffering from incurable diseases. Not surprisingly, he has been very successful in his efforts, much to the gratitude of a large number of people.

My friend had this to say: "Rather than being similar to modern pharmaceutical medicines, this organic germanium compound is more like one of the traditional Chinese medicinal herbs. I have used it to treat a number of different illnesses, and have found its healing effect to be more constitutional than allopathic—that is, it acts on the body as a whole rather than on any specific symptom.

"To put it more simply, your organic germanium cures diseases by inducing the body's own natural healing powers. I am convinced that by increasing the flow of oxygen, organic germanium stimulates latent natural healing powers existing in the human body, thereby resulting in a very effective cure of any illness."

From the way in which various diseases had been cured by organic germanium treatment, I too, had become aware of a rather close link between the action of organic germanium and natural healing processes in the body. However, at that time, I had very little idea of just what these healing powers were, or how they were to be described in scientific terms.

Another interesting visitor came to me some time afterwards, this time an elderly medical practitioner who had become familiar with acupuncture. He told me that the scientific principles behind acupuncture anaesthesia had recently been brought to light, and that more conventional pain suppression anaesthetics, such as morphine etc. will no longer be needed in surgical operations. Furthermore, he continued, patients can be relieved of pain for up to 27 hours and suffer no side-effects. Postoperative progress of the patient also seems far better than after the use of conventional anaesthetics.

In brief, recent research has shown that when acupuncture needles are applied to what are known as *tsubo* in Oriental medicine, the pituitary gland secretes a peptide hormone called beta-endorphin (which consists of 91 amino acids in a 61 to 91 amino acid sequence) resulting in a strong pain-suppressing effect. The *tsubo* vary according to where the operation is to be performed. Three acupuncture needles are inserted precisely at the required positions, and after 15 to 20 minutes the desired anaesthetic effect is achieved. Since the anaesthetic agent is an autogenic anaesthetic produced in the body, there are no undesirable side-effects, and postoperative recovery is rapid. However, the doctor continued to say that since these *tsubo* and other facets of acupuncture are not acknowledged in Western medicine and are not included in university medical courses, this excellent anaesthetic practice is not generally employed.

It dawned on me as I listened that this anaesthetic action is very similar to the action of my organic germanium compound. On being given 3 to 4 grams of organic germanium cancer patients literally writhing in pain have found relief in 15 to 20 minutes. Time and time again, I have witnessed terminal stage cancer patients find release from their torment as if by magic, and be allowed to finally pass from this world in peace.

Pain is a form of warning passed from the troubled area to the brain by means of an electric charge relay mechanism along nerve cells. It is only after this "signal" reaches the brain that we actually feel pain. Anaesthetics, such as morphine, prevent us from feeling pain by interrupting this electric charge relay temporarily by chemical action.

Germanium, on the other hand, was initially thought to interfere with the electric charge relay process due to its semiconductor properties, and this action quite possibly takes place. However, it also seems reasonable that the production of a pseudo-morphine anaesthetic agent called "endorphin" is stimulated in the body by germanium in much the same way as by acupuncture needles. This proposition is certainly supported by the results of experiments on laboratory animals using organic germanium. The color and luster of hormone-secreting organs such as the thyroid and adrenal glands are considerably improved, while the animals' hair becomes glossier, giving the animals a rejuvenated appearance.

In clinical cases, too, germanium has been very effective in the treatment of a number of diseases caused by adrenaline inadequacies, including enlargement of the prostate gland, cancer of the breast and uterine cancer, goiter and uterine myoma, etc. It would thus appear that this germanium compound has a kind of electro-biochemical action quite unlike the effect of conventional pharmaceuticals. For example, germanium increases the amount of oxygen transported by hemoglobin in the red blood cells. The supply of oxygen to tissue cells is thereby increased, resulting in greater cellular activity. This in turn can be assumed to be responsible for various other biochemical processes in relation to cell membrane potential. The pseudo-morphine agent "endorphin" referred to earlier is a peptide hormone secreted from the hypothalamus in the brain, and is thought to be stimulated by the germanium compound.

To think that Oriental medicine that has its origins some 3,000 years ago discovered an anaesthetic procedure, which has now been substantiated by modern science, is exhilarating to say the least! I can only marvel at the wisdom of the ancient Chinese and the systematic development of their knowledge of medicine.

At present, however, the focus of world attention has been turned to the "wonder medication" *interferon*. The existence of this substance was first brought to light more than 20 years ago, and is considered one of the most significant medical discoveries since penicillin, particularly where cancer treatment is concerned. However, just what kind of substance *interferon* is, and how it works, remain very difficult questions to answer.

To put it as briefly as possible, when an infectious virus enters the human body, tissue cells commence to secrete *interferon* (a glycoprotein with a molecular weight of about 40,000) to protect the cells from the viral infection. In addition, there is also an increase in the number of macrophages (one of the leucocytes involved in the removal of malignant tumor cells) for greater effectiveness against cancer cells.

Clinical tests with *interferon* have produced excellent results. So much so that pharmaceutical manufacturers have started to worry that their more conventional products will become obsolete. It should be noted here, however, that *interferon* is not a new drug—it is a substance produced in the human body, whose natural healing powers have been harnessed scientifically.

That famous doctor Robert Koch is quoted as saying, "The best medicines are those substances formed naturally by the human body." It seems he was forecasting the discovery of *interferon*.

Although *interferon* was discovered, and its significance understood, more than 20 years ago, there are several reasons why it has not been used greatly. First, large-scale cell cultures are required which are very difficult to grow. Secondly, since the amount of *interferon* obtained is very small, little has been learned about its chemical structure. Although it has been found to be a glycoprotein, its molecular sequence and its biochemical action in the human body have still not been studied sufficiently. Thirdly, nothing is known about how *interferon* is produced in the cells, and fourthly, *interferon* is unbelievably expensive, one gram costing more than US$100,000.

At present, this wonder-working substance, *interferon*, has still not not been synthesized in the test tube. Only live cells are capable of its production, and furthermore, the only *interferon* which is effective in the human body is that which is produced by human cells.

As the synthesis of *interferon* is practically impossible, and as there seems little likelihood of any suitable method for production being developed in the near future, it has been proposed that the same result might be obtained by somehow inducing the production of *interferon* from living cells in the human body. Consequently, a number of researchers have attempted to force the secretion of *interferon* by stimulating the cells with various toxic substances. However, although this method does in fact stimulate the cells to secrete *interferon*, the stimulating reagents are invariably toxic, and cannot be used for medical purposes.

During my own research, I have often paid attention to matters relating to the electric charge on cell membranes. Apparently the very nature of cancer cells, for example, is changed by alterations in the cellular membrane potential. Nobel prize winner Prof. Albert Szent-Gyorgyi has put forward similar ideas based on electro-biochemical concepts. My germanium compound is an organic compound containing atoms of the semiconductor element germanium. The semiconductor property of the germanium atoms enables this compound to bring about changes in electric charge (as can be seen in the dehydrogenation and super-oxidation effects.)

From the above suppositions, it is postulated that it is this change in membrane potential of the cancer cells that results in the stimulation of *interferon* production. Supporting evidence for this postulation is presented in the accompanying digram.

Throughout this book I have explained the dramatic effects which my organic germanium compound exhibit solely on the basis of an increase in the amount of circulating oxygen in the body. This explanation, however, is inadequate. To be sure, the dehydrogenation effect in the body is certainly an advantage in various medical treatments. However, with the discovery of the induced production of such a powerful weapon as *interferon* in the suppression of diseases and particularly the elimination of cancer cells, I felt an overwhelming sense of conviction that I was moving closer to the truth.

Modern Western medicine is based on an allopathic approach (i.e.,

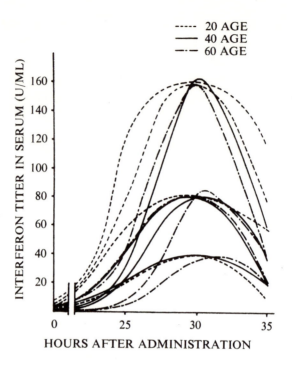

Interferon induction after oral administration of Ge-132 (75 mg/kg) to healthy volunteers.

treating symptoms as each calls for attention.) Cancer-resistant agents are typical examples, but these agents involve undesirable side-effects to a certain extent, resulting in the considerable recent controversy about iatrogenic diseases (diseases caused by medical treatment.)

I think it would be quite proper to call *interferon* a "natural healing substance." In contrast to anticancer agents, *interferon* is produced within the body in order to protect the body from disease. It is designed to support life, and does not, therefore, result in any undesirable side effects in other parts of the body. Furthermore, my organic germanium compound, which induces the production of *interferon*, is also completely nontoxic and free of side-effects. In this sense, it is very similar to traditional Chinese medicines.

Another interesting fact which should be considered here is that just as acupuncture fails to affect some people (i.e., no anaesthetic action) germanium, too, on rare occasions fails to induce the secretion of any quantity of *interferon*. Although the reason is not easy to explain, my observations of clinical cases where organic germanium has been employed tends to make me believe that this phenomenon is due to acidosis of the blood which is a result of loss of a proper acid/alkaline balance.

I would like to state my belief that the induced production and secretion of *interferon* by organic germanium, and of endorphin by acupuncture, establishes a scientific basis for Oriental medicine. Chinese medicinal herbs invariably contain high levels of germanium, and furthermore, it is also possible that these herbs also contain other compounds that induce the production of other interferon-like substances in the body.

In acupuncture, stimulation via the *tsubo* results in the increased production and secretion of endorphin which in turn results in a healing effect. In moxa cautery treatment, the toxic components resulting from the thermal decomposition of protein under the scorched portion of skin are passed into the bloodstream, and subsequently induce the production of *interferon* in the tissue cells.

Both endorphin and *interferon* are types of hormone, each closely related to the other. Living beings have been endowed with these natural healing substances for self-preservation purposes.

I believe future medical treatment will be centered around the use of these and similar substances. The basic concept is expressed as "Sho" in Oriental medicine, "Gesamtheit" in German, and "holistic" in English. On this basis, the amount of circulating oxygen which is so essential to life is increased to strengthen the body's defense against the cause of a disease, and the production of the powerful weapon *interferon* is also increased to join in the fight against the pathogen.

A Prayer for Germanium

"Friends, those who touch this touch humanity"
Walt Whitman, *Leaves of Grass*.

    I have already written thousands of words to describe the efficacy of the organic germanium compound and its background, but feel I have not done it full justice. I have whole-heartedly devoted myself to the study of germanium for close to 30 years. The historical background I have given with many observations I connected and various ideas and thoughts that have occurred to me based on these observations. I am perhaps too eager and too hasty to make public what I have learned about germanium which I am convinced everyone on earth would welcome. In my eagerness perhaps I have written without restraining my own idiosyncrasy before attempting to undertake the necessary steps for the legal and social decorum that are required in publishing novel ideas and unconventional therapeutical means.
    In this connection, I recall a story about a chemist who was asked to analyze a transparent liquid in a test tube to identify it. He immediately made its analysis and reported that the liquid in question consisted of a large quantity of water and a tiny quantity of calcium, sodium and potassium salt. He could not find out that the liquid was actually tears shed by a mother in sorrow.
    At the outset, I intended to describe the therapeutical efficacy of germanium. Gradually, however, I have been led to believe the existence of something in germanium that cannot be fully explained in terms of science in its present stage of development, when I see that obstinate diseases for which modern medicine is powerless are successfully cured by our germanium therapy. Now I consider that the

answer lies in the realm unknowable by science referred to by Alexis Carrel.

I would like to stress the need for modern scientists, particularly medical scientists, to free themselves from the shackles of straitjacketed thought patterns that compel them to be "one-dimensional human beings," and to enter into meditative thinking of higher dimensions. Physicians tend to depend on medical treatises that only represent the surface of a mirror, and fail to see anything through it. All they do is follow what appears on the surface. Such a monodimensional conduct will hardly succeed in saving lives.

Webster's Dictionary defines the word "vision" as "power of perceiving mental images by sharp prophetic sight or rigorous spirit."

Vision should be applied to the study of germanium which must be conducted in a more rigorous manner with thinking on a higher dimensional level than that in other types of research. Only a man who has been captured by the mysterious charm of germanium can succeed in this research. The effort involved is precisely the one needed for realizing a vision. Moreover, there must be careful observation not to overlook any phenomenon that is encountered by filling the mind with the laws of the great universe.

Over the months and years, I have tested organic germanium compound conscientiously, and put it out only with absolute proof based on strict objectivity. In the words of Zen is the expression *saitaku doki* (啐啄同機) which means that when an egg is at the point of hatching, the mother bird and the chick in the egg both peck simultaneously to break the shell, a timing and interaction which demonstrates a marvelous providence in nature. In the same way there is a mysterious *saitaku doki* between the sickness and germanium. When we recognize this wonderful truth and mysterious law in the universe, I believe we can then, for the first time, really understand germanium.

I can only long, night and day, for germanium therapy to become universally available. I deem it advisable to treat organic germanium not as a pharmaceutical but as a means of a therapeutical system which we should build for saving mankind. Germanium has much in common with Chinese medicine, as I have pointed out earlier, and is in harmony with the Oriental medicine, which means that "Natural Therapy Will be Perfected With Germanium."

In closing, I borrow the words of Friedrich Schiller, "The future wavers, but wavering draws on, the present passes swift as an arrow, and the past sinks into the silence of eternity."

Appendix 1

The Organo Germanium Sesquioxide

The compound bis-carboxyethyl germanium sesquioxide and its diamide, bis-carbamylethyl germanium sesquioxide have the following formulae, respectively:

$(GeCH_2CH_2COOH)_2O_3$ and $(GeCH_2CH_2CONH_2)_2O_3$

The compounds bis-carboxyethyl germanium sesquioxide and bis-carbamylethyl germanium sesquioxide are prepared as illustrated by the following equations:

$GeHCl_3 + CH_2\text{: }CHCN \longrightarrow Cl_3Ge\text{-}CH_2CH_2CN$

$Cl_3Ge\text{-}CH_2CH_2CN \longrightarrow Cl_3GeCH_2CH_2COOH$
$\nearrow$
Hydrolyze

$Cl_3GeCH_2CH_2COOH + SOCl_2 - Cl_3GeCH_2CH_2COCl$

$2Cl_3GeCH_2CH_2COCl \longrightarrow (GeCH_2CH_2COOH)_2O_3$
$\nearrow$
Hydrolyze

or,
$2Cl_3GeCH_2CH_2COCl \longrightarrow (GeCH_2CH_2CONH_2)_2O_3$
$\nearrow$
Ammonia water

The process of making the compounds is as follows: β-cyanothyl-trichlorogermanium (trichloro-germanium ethylene cyanide) is obtained by the action of acrylonitrile on the known compound trichloro-germanium (germanium chloroform). β-cyanoethyltrichlorogermanium is converted into β-trichloro-germanium propionic acid (trichloro-

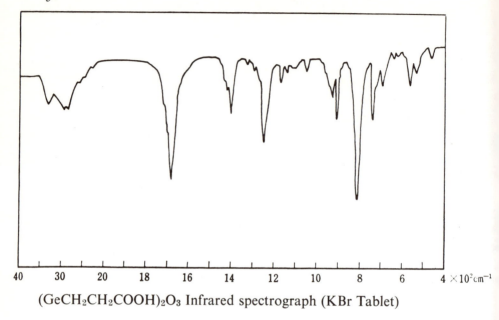

$(GeCH_2CH_2COOH)_2O_3$ Infrared spectrograph (KBr Tablet)

germanium propionic acid) by hydrolysis in the presence of a mineral acid and by the action of thionylchloride. This latter compound is converted to trichlorogermanium propionyl chloride. Hydrolysis of this compound with water produces bis-carboxyethyl germanium sesquioxide. By the action of ammonia water on trichlorogermanium propionyl chloride, bis-carbamylethyl germanium sesquioxide is produced.

Appendix 2

2-1 On Acute Toxicity of Organo Germanium

Examination was made on LD_{50} of organic germanium on rats and mice.

1. *Methods* Germanium used in the experiment was bis-carboxyethyl germanium sesquioxide. Since it has a low saturation point, the sample was used in the form of a suspension which was prepared with 0.5% carboxymethyl cellose.

2. *Animals:* Animals used in the experiment were Wistar strain rats weighing 150 g$\pm$20 g and I.C.R. strain mice of 20 g$\pm$5 g in weight. In both rats and mice, 20 animals or 10 males and 10 females formed one group for experiment.

They were raised on pellet feeds (Nippon Korea KK CE-2) at a constant room temperature and humidity of 24°C$\pm$2°C and 50% $\pm$5%, respectively. Water was supplied *ad libitum* by water bottles.

The presence of toxicity was determined on the 7th day after administration. The liquid amounts of administration to the animals were 10 ml/kg (rats) and 40 ml/kg (mice, 0.4 ml/10 g).

3. *Experimental Results*

A. ORAL ADMINISTRATION TO RATS

LD_{50} of germanium on rats by oral administration was as given below.

♂ 10 g/kg<
♀ 10 g/kg<

General Toxic Symptoms: In a dosage level of 5,000–10,000 mg/kg, no acceleration or depression of voluntary movements, lowering of reactions to stimulus or any other external symptoms (such as abnormality in movements or reflection were observed. Thus, no toxic symptoms worthy of particular attention were noted.

Table 1. Results of Oral Administration to Both Sexes of Rats and Mice

Sex Dosage mg/kg	♂ ♀ Days of observation 1, 2, ... 7		LD_{50}
5,000	0/10→	0/10	
8,000	0/10→	0/10	10 g/kg<
10,000	0/10→	0/10	
LD_{50}	10 kg/kg<		

As the dosage was 1 ml/100 g due to the hard soluble properties of germanium, the animals indicated signs of disagreeable feeling when the drug was administered. However, it is considered that this symptom is not produced by germanium compound.

B. ORAL ADMINISTRATION TO MICE

LD_{50} of germanium on mice by oral administration was as given below.

♂ 10 g/kg<
♀ 10 g/kg<

General Toxic Symptoms: In a dosage level of 5,000–10,000 mg/kg, no effect of administration was observed on voluntary movements, reactions or any other external behavior.

Anatomical Findings on both Sexes of Rats and Mice after Seven

Days of Administration: Gross anatomical observation of liver, kidneys, spleen and other organs exhibited no noteworthy changes. However, soft feces of transient nature appeared within 24 hours after administration, although their relationship with germanium was not established.

Table 2 LD_{50} of Germanium by Oral Administration.

	Sex	LD_{50}
Rats Wistar	♂ ♀	10 g/kg< 10 g/kg<
Mice I.C.R.	♂ ♀	10 g/kg< 10 g/kg<

Results: The following results were obtained as LD_{50} of organic germanium on rats and mice.

From the above results it may be concluded that this organo germanium possesses practically no toxic properties.

2-2 On Chronic Toxicity of Organo Germanium

Germanium was orally administered to rats daily for six consecutive months to study the possible toxicity of germanium.
Material and Method
1. *Material*
   Germanium used for experiment was bis-carboxyethyl germanium sesquioxide. Since it has a low saturation point in water, the sample was used in the form of a suspension prepared by 0.5% carboxymethyl cellulose.
2. *Method*
1) Experimental Groups
   From among the rats thus raised, 40 males and 40 females of well-grown animals were obtained. These animals were divided into four

control groups of 10 each, control, 30 mg/kg, 300 mg/kg and 300 mg/kg. The germanium preparation was introduced into the stomach through an oral tube.

2) Items Examined

a. General Symptoms

Observation for possible changes in behavior, hair, etc. was made during the administration.

b. Measurement of Body Weight

All animals were weighed every three days.

c. Hematological Findings

The blood collected from the pulmonary artery of the heart at autopsy was examined to get the following data:

The number of erythrocytes

The amount of hemoglobin (the cyanmethemoglobin method)

Hematocrit value (the capillary method)

The number of leucocytes

The differential count of leucocytes

d. Examination of Various Functions

Serum was separated from blood samples collected from the pulmonary artery of the heart at autopsy to test the followings:

serum G. O. T. (Reitman-Frankel method)

serum G. P. T. (Reitman-Frankel method)

serum alkaline phosphatase (Bessey-Lowry method)

serum cholesterol

serum urinary nitrogen (Indophenol method)

serum total protein (Semi-micro-Kjeldahl method)

blood sugar (Enzyme method)

A/G ratio (the cataphoresis method with the use of cellulose acetate films)

serum electrolysis Na^+, K^+ (the flame method)

e. Measurement of Weight of Various Organs and Histopathological Examination.

The wet weight of principal organs was measured at each autopsy. Histological examination was made by providing H. E. stain upon fixation with a 10% buffer formalin solution on the cerebrum (including the cerebellium), pituitary gland, lungs liver, spleen, kidneys,

kidneys, pancreas, duodenum, seminal glands, prostate glands, overies, uterus, thyroid glands and bone marrow.
Results
Results
1. General Symptoms
   None of the groups exhibited emaciation, or coarse lusterless hair. Nor were abnormalities observed in general symptoms.
2. Change in Body Weight
   Each group indicated a trend of normal gain in body weight and showed no difference from control gain at the end of the administration period.
3. Mortality Rate
   All animals survived throughout the experimental period.
4. In the 30 mg/kg group, 300 mg/kg group and 3,000 mg/kg group, neither sex showed any particular abnormalities.
   However, in the 300 mg/kg group and 3,000 mg/kg group, two male rats, respectively, gained an unusually high value of leukocytes, but it was pathologically determined that those were caused by bronchopneumonia, and had no relation to the administration of germanium compound.
5. Examination of Various Functions
   In the 30 mg/kg group and 3,000 mg/kg group, neither males nor females showed any particular abnormalities.
6. Weight of Organs
   In neither of the sexes in any of the groups, were particular abnormalities detected.
7. Pathological Findings
(1) Gross Findings
   Gross pathological examination revealed no abnormalities in any of the organs. Although pneumonia was found in some animals, it had nothing to do with the administration of the germanium compound.
(2) Microscopic Findings
   Picture 1 to picture 18, revealed no sign of toxicity in any of the organs.

Discussion

Oral administration of germanium to both sexes of rats at a daily dose of 3,000 mg/kg for six months did not cause even a single death nor abnormalities in external appearances or body weight curves. Therefore, the germanium compound is considered to have a very low toxicity.

Conclusion

Oral administration of germanium to both sexes of rats on a daily dose of 3,000 mg/kg for six months, caused neither inhibition of body weight gain nor abnormalities in the blood, or in the function of various organs; nor did the weight of organs, gross findings or microscopic findings show any particular anomaly.

2-3 Experiment on Possible Deformity-inducing Properties of Germanium

Effects on Rat Fetuses

Examination has been conducted on possible deformity-inducing effects of germanium on rat fetuses by administering the drug to pregnant Wistar rats.

Material and Method
1. Drug

Germanium, a water-insoluble white powder, was used in suspension in a 1% CMC solution.

2. Experimental Animals

Wistar rats 80 to 90 days old were used. To obtain pregnant animals, nulliparous rats were mated to males of the same strain by keeping them in couples through the night. The Oriental Ration NMF was fed and water in bottles was given to the animals. Experiment was conducted at a constant temperature of $23°C \pm 2°C$ and a constant humidity of $55\% \pm 5\%$.

3. Administration Method

The drug was orally administered for 7 days from the 7th day of pregnancy.

4. Dosage

Three levels of dosage were employed: 400 mg/kg, 200 mg/kg and

5 mg/kg. A 1% CMC solution in the amount of 1 ml/100 g was given to the control.

Results and Discussion

1) Effects on Mother's Body

In each group, the body weight up to the day of abdominal incision indicated no significant difference from the control.

2) Effects on Fetuses

No difference was noted between the control and each administration group in the average number of implantation per litter, number of absorbed fetuses and number of live fetuses. However, in the average body weight of fetuses, there was a significant difference of $P<0.05$ between the control and the 200 mg/kg administration group: the gain of the control group was 5.6 g$\pm$0.40 g whereas that for the latter was 5.24 g$\pm$0.40 g. A significant difference ($P<0.01$) was also observed with the 400 mg/kg administration group which indicated a gain of 4.10 g$\pm$0.50 g. The group with the large dose presented a case of immature growth (normal macination).

Skeletal abnormalities: The control group showed 5 cases (2.3%) of abnormalities (in all 5 cases one rib of either the left or the right side was missing), whereas in the 5 mg/kg administration group there were 3 cases (1.69%), and the 200 mg/kg administration group 4 cases (1.90%) including 3 cases of missing ribs and 1 case of abnormal lumbar.

In the 400 mg/kg administration group, 3 cases of missing ribs, 1 case of asymmetrical ossification centers of the breastbone and 1 case of incomplete growth of the parietal bone, breast bone, and lumbar bone were found.

3) Effects on Newborn

Natural delivery was obtained from 3 rats of each group. In this experiment, the ratio of absorbed fetuses was 6.3% for the 5 mg/kg administration group, 9.8% for the 200 mg/kg administration group and 20.6% for the 4000 mg/kg administration group as compared with 0% for the control. As a result of Chi^2-examination, a significant difference ($p<0.01$) was noted in the 4000 mg/kg administration group. In addition, with respect to the average body weight at birth, a significant decrease in body weight gain was observed in the 200 mg/kg group within a risk ratio of 5% and in the 4000 mg/kg group within a risk ratio of 1%. However, as far as the body weight gain up to 3 weeks after birth is concerned, although the 4000 mg/kg group presented some decrease in the average body weight, none of the cases represented any significant difference. As regards sex ratio, lactation ratio and abnormalities (their location), no difference was noted between the control and each administration group.

Summary

(1) In both the control and the administration groups, no effect of the drug was observed with respect to general condition of the pregnant body or maintenance of pregnancy.

(2) Examination in the last stages of pregnancy revealed some significant difference in the number of implantations between the control and the large dose group. Otherwise, no difference was detected in abnormal organs, sex ratio or lactation ratio.

Index

A
abdominal adhesion, 79
abdominal dropsy, 79, 80, 86
acid/alkaline, 151
acidification, 89
acidosis, 151
acupuncture, 146, 151
acupuncturist, 33
acute toxicity, 159
adrenal glands, 68, 91
agony, 73
alveolar pyorrhea, 85
amyloidosis, 52
anaesthetic effect, 146
anasarca, 58
anatomical findings, 160
angina pectoris, 70, 71
aplastic anemia, 97
apoplexy, 62, 64
articular rheumatism, 56, 75, 77
arteriosclerosis, 70, 71
asphyxiation, 64
asthma, 15, 78, 79
atopic dermatitis, 57
autogenic anaesthetic, 146
autonomic ataxia, 77

B
balanced diet, 14, 41
Bardeen, 18
Behcet, 61
Behcet's syndrome, 97

beta-endorphin, 146
birth of healthy life, 44
bis-carboxyethyl, 159
black cataracts, 65
bladder, 15, 76
blocked bile duct, 85
blood viscosity, 103
bone tumor, 120
brain, 109
brain cells, 84
brain hemorrhage, 70
brain tumor, 124
Brattain, 18
breast, 15, 70
breast cancer, 67
bronchial asthma, 56
bronchitis, 81
burns, 74

C
cadmium, 81, 83
calcareous deposit, 82
Canada, 49
cancer, 70, 99, 101, 126, 130
cancer cells, 99
cancer of the breast, 147
cancer of the larynx, 114
cancer of the liver, 122
cancer of the lung, 15
Cancer Ward, 24
carbon monoxide, 64
carbon monoxide poisoning, 36

carboxy methyl cellose, 159
cardiac infarction, 76
cardiac insufficiency, 15
Carrel, Alexis, 36, 125, 133, 135
cartilage malignancy, 109
cellular oxygen deficiency, 99
cerebral apoplexy, 70
cerebellar degeneration, 59
cerebral thrombosis, 75, 92
cervical tumor, 70
chalazion, 72
chemistry, 139
chilblains, 85
Chinese medicinal herbs, 145, 151
cholecystitis, 72
chronic asthma, 97
chronic rheumatism, 70
chronic toxicity, 161
cirrhosis, 85
Clarit, 21
climacteric disorders, 70
constipation, 56, 79, 140
contaminated food, 84
convalescence, 74
corns, 74
cure, 75
cure reaction, 74, 75
cystitis, 72

D

deceptive phenomenon, 75
dehydrogenating, 103
dehydrogenation, 97
depression, 70
depressive psychosis, 92, 93, 94, 95
detached retinas, 65
diabetes, 15, 80
diabetes mellitus, 79
diarrhea, 81
difficulty in walking, 89
divination, 140

dosage, 75
dropsical swelling, 79
dry cough, 104
Durit, 21

E

eczemas, 74
edema, 58
effects on animals, 34
Einstein, 32
ekasilicon, 18
electronics industry, 141
elixir of life, 51
empyema, 85
endorphin, 147, 151
enervation, 69
epilepsy, 70
esophageal varices, 79
eye diseases, 65

F · G

festering wounds, 126
gastric ulcer, 80, 81
gastritis, 80
germanium bathing, 139
germanium sesquioxide, 159
German measles, 85
Gesamtheit, 151
ginseng, 25, 26
gland cancer, 70
glands, 67
glaucoma, 65
glycoprotein, 148
goiter, 147
gout, 56
Guillain-Barre-Syndrome, 86
Gyorgyi, Albert Szent, 150

H

hardness of hearing, 76
headaches, 79
heart troubles, 70

heavy metal, 84
hematemesis, 75
hepatic cirrhosis, 15
hepatic dysfunction, 62
hepatitis, 97
hepatoma, 59
herpes, 74
Herrigel, Eugen, 31
hives, 56
Honda-Fujishima, 23
holistic, 151
hypersensitivity, 79
hypertension, 15, 66, 71, 79
hyperthyroidism, 81
hypodermic injections, 131
hysteria, 91

I
iatrogenic diseases, 150
infantile asthma, 85
infantile nephritis, 85
inflammation of maxillary sinus, 15
influenza, 85, 89
insomnia, 79, 140
interferon, 148, 150, 151
International Angiological Congress, 65
intestinal disorders, 56
itching eruptions, 69
itches, 79
Iwanami Publishers, 139

J · K · L
Japan Pathological Society, 52
Japan Society for Cancer Therapy, 103
Keio University hospital, 118
kidney, 56, 79, 109
kidney cancer, 134
Koch, Robert, 148
languor, 69

larynx, 15
leukemia, 15, 118, 121
ligated circle of Willis, 84
limbs, 69
Lindbergh, 133
liver, 56, 79, 84, 91, 109
liver abcesses, 126
liver cancer, 104
liver cirrhosis, 79, 80
liver function, 80
liver tumor, 86
Lourdes, 125
low blood pressure, 140
lumbago, 79
lung, 84, 104
lung cancer, 100, 104, 106, 107, 109, 132
lymphatic metastasis, 70

M
macrophages, 148
Madam Curie, 20
malignant tumor, 70
manic-depressive psychosis, 91
Man, the Unknown, 36
medical tribune, 99
medulla, 82
melena, 75
menstrual pains, 77
mental disease, 90
mental disorder, 76
mercury, 81, 82
mercury poisoning, 81
metamorphic rock, 138
miracle waters, 133
mongolism, 85
moxa cautery, 151
muscular atrophy, 85
myelogenous leukemia, 118, 119
myocardial infarction, 70
myoma, 68
myoma of the uterus, 15

N · O

nephrosis syndrome, 58
nervous overstrain, 89
neuralgia, 15, 140
neurosis, 15
Newsweek, 134
Noguchi, Hideyo, 117
nystagmus, 59
odor, 74
organo germanium sesquioxide, 157
oriental medicine, 146
osteitis, 126
otitis media, 85
oxygen consumption of the brain, 91
oxygen deficiency, 14, 15, 89, 91
oxygen deficit, 48

P

pain, 101
PB report, 20
PCB, 84
piles, 75
pneumonia, 78, 81, 89, 97
Poincaré, Jules Henri, 15
poisoning, 64
poisonous matter, 97
polybiphenyl chloride, 84
poor circulation, 140
positive-hole effect, 19
post-operative treatment of cancer, 70
pregnancy, 43
prevention of metastasis, 103
proper acid-basebalance, 14
prostate, 67
prostate gland, 68, 69, 105, 147
prostate gland cancers, 104
pyelitis, 72

R

Raynaud's disease, 64, 70, 71
religion, 140
Reppe, 31
retinal disorder, 44
retrobulbar neuritis, 57
rice plants, 27
ringing in the ears, 145
Ronninghof, 115
Rumania, 106

S

sarcoidosis, 95
Sato, Haruo, 103
Schrodinger, 29
schizophrenia, 77
sclerotic heart, 71
seizure, 87, 88
Selye, Hans, 49, 50, 100
semiconductors, 102
senile mental diseases, 70
sequela of cerebral apoplexy, 70
sequela to apoplesy, 70
Sho, 151
Shockley, 18
skin, 73
skin lesion, 126
SMON, 58, 97
softening of the brain, 15, 70, 91, 92
Solzhenitsyn, Alexander, 24
apleen tumor, 86
splinters, 74
stiffness, 81
stomach, 56, 71
stomach ulcer, 70, 71, 72, 75
stools, 69
stress, 49
Subacute myelo-optico-neuropathy, 58

T
Tanak, Takahiro, 69, 92
thrombosis, 70
tinnitus, 59
tofu, 107
Tohoku University, 103
Tokyo University hospital, 119, 125
toothache, 85
toxic elements, 56
toxicity, 55
toxicity tests, 35
toxic symptoms, 160
transistors, 141
tsubo, 146, 151
tubercular peritonitis, 126
tuberculosis of the bones, 126

U · V · W
University of Montreal, 49
unpolished rice, 107
uterus, 68
uterine cancer, 67, 147
uterine myoma, 67, 147
Vitrit, 21
Voronkov, 139
Waltenburg, 100
Warburg method, 38
Warburg, Otto, 99
warts, 74
water in bottles of water, 164
Water of Life, 119
water of lourdes, 134
Webster's dictionary, 154
whiplash injury, 91
whiplash syndrome, 77
white cataracts, 97
white sugar, 107
winkler, 18
World Congress of Natural Medicine, 96

Y · Z
Yamabuki-no-omizu, 136
Zen, 154